Journeys in

June 2012

Journeys in Cancerland

John-Peter Bradford

Lisa Newman

Foreword by Sholom Glouberman

Health and Everything Publications
Toronto, Ontario

Printed in the United States

ISBN 978-0-9812618-2-9 (paperback)

☉

Library and Archives Canada Cataloguing in Publication

Bradford, J.P., Newman, L.
Journeys in Cancerland / John-Peter Bradford, Lisa Newman.

ISBN 978-0-9812618-2-9

CIP subject topics forthcoming

CIP reference numbers forthcoming

Contents

Foreword

This book contains two object lessons in patient participation. For a long time, patients barely participated in their own care. Once diagnosed with a disease like cancer, they would enter an all-consuming acute care system that took over their lives until they went into remission or they died. That this is no longer true is due, for the most part, to patients and caregivers like John-Peter Bradford and Lisa Newman who have begun to take charge of their care. Their stories are not merely instructive about cancer care – they are lessons in how to live with life threatening illness and how to face death.

These stories are particularly meaningful for the Patients' Association of Canada because they provide an opportune context for understanding how our all-consuming acute care system came to be, and how and why it has begun to change.

Modern healthcare systems began with the rise of "scientific medicine" in the late 19th century. The major killers at the time of Robert Koch and Louis Pasteur were infectious diseases such as anthrax, tuberculosis, and typhoid fever. They were the first to identify the microorganisms that cause such disease and then to develop vaccines to prevent them. The recognition that many major causes of death could be identified and cured spurred the professionalization of physicians, the construction of the acute care hospital, and other elements of modern health systems: rigorous experimental science, replicable testing, definitive treatment protocols, and research on prevention.

Because most infectious diseases are clearly identifiable, there is little or no ambiguity or uncertainty that might require patients to be engaged. Once this paradigm was established in the early 20th century, the typical patients gave their bodies over to the system and, once admitted to the hospital, contributed little or nothing to their treatment. The hope was that all diseases would ultimately be dealt with in this way.

The modern healthcare system was enormously successful. Between 1900 and 1970, the diseases that killed us shifted from being acute infectious diseases to long term chronic ones. Today, comparatively few deaths result from acute infectious diseases. Instead, the vast majority result from chronic conditions with multiple causes, long periods of onset, and episodic acute events.

The course of chronic disease is far more ambiguous than acute illness. It can vary considerably from one person to another and in the same person from one time to another. Medical intervention is only one aspect of managing a chronic condition; it also depends on many other factors including the patients themselves. We have come to see that cancer is not a single acute disease but is made up of a large number of chronic conditions, only some of which are life threatening. Most importantly, we have come to see that patients have a large role to play in dealing with the disease. At the Patients' Association of Canada, we think that they also have a critical role to play in redesigning the care services they receive and in making the system of care more patient-sensitive.

These two stories are excellent examples of how people have begun to take charge of their care. John-Peter Bradford's story comments extensively on the system and brings a matter-of-fact directness to understanding the disease he faces and how to respond to it. Lisa Newman had to relive some of her experience with grief and loss to tell the story of her husband's struggle with the disease and his death. She very much wanted to help other family members in similar circumstances and so she works at articulating the lessons from her experience. The result is a practical and comprehensive guide that will be indispensible for all caregivers.

Sholom Glouberman, PhD
President, Patients' Association of Canada

Cancer: An Unexpected Gift

John-Peter Bradford

Part One

What a Trip!

I am a cancer survivor. I am writing this because I want you to champion the development of new forms of support for cancer patients, caregivers, and healthcare professionals. Cancer is becoming more widespread, so the need for support will only increase.

Many patients go through hell. Family and friends who care for them have to learn to do so without help while their emotional and physical lives are being disrupted. Healthcare professionals like doctors and nurses are often pushed to their limits. They all need help.

I'm going to illustrate why and how by telling you the story of my cancer journey. Actually, I hate the term "cancer journey," but I'm using it. Almost every other writer does. I don't know why, but I do know that cancer isn't a trip that I'd sign up to take, nor is it an adventure that I'd wish anyone to experience.

But before I tell you my story, let me introduce myself. I live in Ottawa, Ontario. My wife and I run a small consulting company. We are very happily married, with a blended family consisting of three adult children and three small grandchildren. My cancer was a surprise. When the first symptoms appeared, I was living a healthy, full life and felt great. I exercised regularly, ate well, played music and sports, and was active in the community. My wife, Annie, and I supported each other, as she too had a vibrant and varied life apart from our business, including significant volunteer commitments. I soon discovered that our marriage not only prepared me well for the daunting frustrations and various tests that having cancer threw at me, but also was my salvation. Annie was a calm, nurturing, steadfast – and essential – support throughout the cancer experience. We faced my disease together, just as we had faced the challenges of living and working together and dealt with the complications and vagaries of merging two families. Our children were teenagers when we married!

I was tempted to call this piece "how I went from a perfunctory visit to the doctor to losing half of my neck to cancer, while coming to grips with fear, family, meaning in life, the healthcare system, and my mortality." But, I won't; it might give away too much of the story.

You'd think that I would have dealt with many of those things before. For example, when I underwent heart by-pass journey and recovered from it. The heart surgeon gave me 96%+ odds of complete recovery, however, so I really didn't feel that threatened. I called my initial and only symptom a stitch because it only happened when I was running. I found it odd, as it was in my lower chest – rather high for a stitch. My family doctor discovered my heart problem when I described the stitch to her. I was scheduled to play basketball that evening. From my description, she strongly suspected that I had a heart problem. She asked me to stay to discuss the situation and in very clear terms ordered me not to play basketball or exercise until the diagnosis was confirmed. I told her I was late for a game, and since she didn't know for sure, I'd play but take it easy.

She called Annie, my wife, who was in the waiting room. They blocked the door until I agreed not to play that evening.

My stupid macho behaviour notwithstanding, I found it very hard to believe that I was sick. Generally, I felt fine. I played basketball or ran five out of seven days a week. I didn't smoke, didn't drink much, and ate a healthy diet. I had no chest or arm pains, no shortness of breath, none of the other warning signs of heart disease.

After that appointment with my GP, everything happened very quickly. In a few days, I was diagnosed with "left main disease," a.k.a. the widow maker, a blockage of the artery that delivers 70% of the heart's blood supply. The danger was clear. A heart attack would have cut off that blood supply and I would have died. But, they caught the problem in time and I had emergency surgery. Before the operation, the surgeon assured me that apart from my heart problem, I had the fitness level of an athlete; this augured well for a good surgical outcome. He gave me a 96% chance of full recovery and assured me that although it would hurt like hell, I would recover. The doctor was right. After surgery, I felt like I'd been mauled by a monster; I felt very vulnerable physically and emotionally. The steps to recovery were very clearly laid out by the Heart Institute staff. It was a job that I went about methodically, walking just a bit more than the prescribed distance every day, resting, reading, and keeping my mind in shape. Soon, I was working, exercising, and even playing basketball again.

Please don't get me wrong. I required (and received) wonderful support from my wife, other family members, and friends during recovery.

Emotionally, I was humbled. I was grateful for the help I received from others and I was determined to get better. The recovery was physically challenging. But, despite the initial shock and trepidation, I was never deeply afraid. Perhaps this was because my by-pass happened quickly (I had the by-pass within two weeks of first seeing my GP). I was also a textbook case: the characteristics of my heart disease were well known, and the treatment was straightforward, though it did include a five hour major surgery. My prognosis was extremely good, and I was in the hands of one of the best surgeons in Canada. The risks were minimal; the outcome was virtually certain.

Facing Fear

I was scared stiff at the start of my cancer journey.

In stark contrast to the by-pass situation, my cancer diagnosis was not clear-cut. It took a long time to get a definitive diagnosis and even longer to start treatment. The risks were considerable and the outcome was not certain, even though my oncologists were the best in their fields. The survival numbers are improving – in some cases dramatically – but, on average, cancer is still more likely than not to be a killer, or a "life-shortener". No matter what a doctor tells you, or how consoling people are, the prospect of having cancer is frightening.

As a child, I was terribly afraid of dying. Sometimes, the fear was overwhelming. Once, when I was about six, I panicked in the middle of a John Wayne movie and ran out of the theatre. My aunt, who had taken me to the movie, caught up to me and asked what was wrong. Even though my heart was pounding, I was too ashamed to own up to my fear. I told her that my stomach was sore and snuggled up for a consoling hug. Over the years, the fear subsided. After my reaction to by-pass surgery, I thought the fear was gone or at least reduced to the odd manageable twinge – a raw nerve that was only hit once every few years and then only briefly.

But, I was wrong. I was terrified that the cancer would kill me and I was afraid to die. I was also frightened that I would put my wife through a hellish caregiving experience that would end in loss for her. I was afraid and ashamed that I might be a coward throughout the process. And I was frightened that I would be a bad example for my children – that I would lose my identity in the health care system and that I would be so consumed by the disease that I would forget about living.

For a day or two, I was an emotional and psychological wreck, alternating between paralysis, numbness, and panic. Very quickly, however, I realized how dysfunctional that was. I had to do something to change.

I tried every calming and relaxing technique I knew. I also remembered how some friends and relatives approached their deaths. I had had long conversations and had been intimately involved with some of them as they approached their ends. Those who died calmly and at peace shared these characteristics: they accepted and focused exactly on the reality they were living, they paid attention to the well-being of significant others in their lives, and they delighted in simple pleasures. They changed what they could and accepted what they couldn't.

These reflections – and the love of my wife – helped me first to accept my situation and then to deal with it calmly, methodically, and even joyfully. My focus changed from "poor me" to gratitude for the help I was getting from my wife and others. I focused too on helping my caretakers as best I could. I stopped railing at things beyond my control and began to become a responsible patient, living as fully as I could.

In a strange way, I was enjoying life. I found myself actually living my answers to a number of big questions: What is mortality and how do I come to grips with it? What does it mean to live a good life? What is good health care if you're on the receiving end? What are my responsibilities to others? How does one transform fear into a positive emotion? Answering the questions by observing and reflecting on my actions was very rewarding.

Instead of my emotions holding me back, they fired me up. This wasn't as difficult as it may seem. The possibility of death or surgical maiming focused me. I *needed* to be clear-headed and emotionally clean; so, I needed to transform the negative emotions to positive motivation. I found it helpful to deal with my daily challenges head-on, thoroughly, factually, putting one foot in front of the other, reflecting on the journey as it unfolded.

Some friends said that I was being courageous. I didn't see it that way, but I did see real courage in other patients who dealt with situations far more dire than mine. Many had hopeless diagnoses – some were bereft of adequate support systems, others were single parents of young children, for many the disease put them in nearly impossible financial situations, others had to travel long distances to get treatment, still others made lifestyle and social changes on a massive scale . . . and on and on.

My wife called my approach "Zen-like." She was right in the sense that it wasn't emotionally indulgent. I simply faced my fears, expressed my emotions, and got on with dealing with my plight.

The key, for me, was accepting my situation. Surprisingly quickly, my feelings became positive. I felt good about living life as fully as possible, cherishing moments with family and friends, and being an actively engaged partner with my caregivers. I accepted the inevitability of my death, even the possibility that I would die of this cancer. That said, I worked hard to prevent that from happening (even as I realized I couldn't control the outcome). Through that simple act of acceptance, I found that coming to grips with mortality and my fears wasn't such a big deal. For me, it required focusing on what was in front of me, remembering to love and accept the love of others, living as fully possible, finding joy and wonder in little things. Those simple things, for which I had longed for much of my life, now came with relative ease.

I worked diligently to become an active, informed partner in my treatment. I didn't want to become infantilized by the health care system like many people, including some who were very close to me. It's easy to be intimidated by the aura of authority and all-knowing invincibility surrounding doctors, especially when you don't really understand your disease or treatment and are, in a very real sense, dependent upon them and other caregivers. I refused to simply check my brain at the clinic door, to stop thinking, to lose my curiosity, to stop looking for information and evidence related to my disease, and to become a passive recipient of medical care.

I wanted an informed and emotionally clean partnership with my doctors and other healthcare providers. Luckily, I wound up with oncologists who welcomed that. As I mention in more detail later, this was vitally important . . . for more than one reason.

Telling the Story

My story is told in a series of emails and reflections that I wrote during the cancer journey (the one exception is the first email in this piece, which is from my wife to me). The emails began as notes to my wife and close family members. As people heard that I was sick, they would write or call to ask how I was. In response, I simply added them to the email list. In the end, more than 50 people were receiving the emails, and the emails themselves had become more elaborate.

I have not changed a word in the emails. They are exactly as I wrote them. I think that they tell a better story that way.

Writing the emails was therapeutic. It forced me to face my situation with sustained discipline, focus, and clarity of thought. In many ways, it became the most meaningful and emotionally compelling job I had ever had. Although the emails were about me and my disease, researching and writing them took me out of myself. They took on a life of their own and my center of attention became what I was learning and for whom I was writing. An added benefit was that I became more and more sophisticated about things medical, which made me a better, more responsible partner for my doctors as well as more attuned to the obligations of healthcare providers.

In contrast to the emails, my reflections below are not real time observations, although they began as such. They have been edited, changed, and crafted for this piece.

Diagnosis: September 2008 to February 2009

I went to see my GP about a smallish lump in my neck. At first, I had thought it was a sign of an infection, a simple swollen gland. The problem was that I didn't feel sick; I didn't have a fever or any other symptoms, but the lump wasn't going away. My GP prescribed an antibiotic and said that if the lump didn't go away after treatment, then we'd have to look for other explanations, like a cyst, benign growth, blocked salivary gland, or cancer. She ordered an ultra-sound of my neck and an x-ray of my neck and chest to see if there were any other obvious problems.

Email Received October 30, 2008 – from my wife, Annie

John-Peter

Your x-ray results show no abnormalities, evidence of the by-pass surgery and your lungs are clear. Our GP's assistant took me next door and we read the report together. She promised to give the report to the doctor when she comes in today. I told her the lump has not disappeared yet, even after taking the antibiotics. She told me to have you come in to see the doctor again if you are still worried. The fastest route is to see a doctor whose specialty is General Otolaryngology (ear, nose and throat) at the ENT clinic (Module "O") at the General. Our family doctor set up an appointment there on Monday at 2PM. The ENT doctor will do a fine needle biopsy.

When my GP received the ultra-sound report on the lump in my neck and considered the speed with which it had enlarged, she broke down doors at the Ottawa Hospital to get the biopsy done quickly. She was fairly certain that there was a cancer, which is why she acted so quickly.

I acted quickly, too, as precaution. Assuming the diagnosis was cancer, I knew the importance of a speedy diagnosis and treatment plan. I would probably need a good oncologist.

Email Sent December 2, 2008

The result is that there is no conclusive result!! The biopsy needs to be re-done; they need more cellular material to make a diagnosis. One problem with fine needle biopsies is that they take so little material. The doctor is literally drawing cells from the tumor through a very skinny needle. The procedure doesn't get many cells. Additionally, if the needle isn't inserted in to a cancerous region of a tumor, the result can indicate no cancer when there is cancer. This is called a false negative. The next procedure will happen next Monday; results will be fast-tracked. Mysteriously, he will do more fine needle aspirations. Frustrating and a pain in the ass, er, neck.

Email Sent December 16, 2008

After a couple of months of tests to see if a lump in my neck is cancerous, I still have no definitive answer.

The lump is big – about the size of an egg lying sideways and protruding a bit from my neck, right under the mandibular joint in the jawbone. The CT scan images show it to be fairly large inside, too. Pain is sporadic – mostly when I move my head in a way that presses on the lump, but there is a constant dull throbbing. This makes it difficult to sing or play basketball, perhaps a small mercy for the choir I sometimes join and my basketball teammates.

Since October, I have undergone a complete blood work-up, x-rays of my neck and chest, ultra-sound of my neck, five fine needle aspiration (FNA) biopsy samples taken in two batches (2 samples the first time; 3 the second) and a CT scan of my neck.

The ultra-sound and CT results are the same: could be cancer, could be benign. In both cases, FNA was recommended.

The doctor also examined my throat with a scope and found no irregularities or cells that look suspicious. Again this appears hopeful, but he cautioned that it was only a visual diagnosis, and therefore imprecise. As he said, "I've done this before, concluded there was no cancer, and been wrong."

So, the next step is to remove the tumor and biopsy the whole thing. This will be done on a priority basis, I hope before Christmas. The surgeon, former Chief of Otolaryngology (ear, nose and throat) at the Ottawa Hospital, will do the honours. I will also have an abdominal ultra-sound to check for other possible cancer sites.

Even though they had not found any cancer cells, the results of the biopsies were inconclusive. This meant little in itself, however, since FNA biopsies, although accurate when they find a positive (i.e., cancerous) result, are also notorious for returning false negatives. The needles are relatively thin and can miss malignant portions of a tumor and simply penetrate swollen tissue instead.

The FNA is the weakest biopsy test that can be done in these circumstances. The high rate of false negatives makes me wonder why this test is done at all. Even more confusing: why is it done a second or third time after inconclusive results, especially in cases like mine where many signs were pointing to cancer? The procedure doesn't take much time, but scheduling an FNA and waiting for the results sometimes takes weeks. Surely, this gives undetected cancers time to grow and get worse and also causes anxiety and fear in patients. The alternative is an excisional biopsy where a part of the tumor is cut out (excised) and then examined for cancer. This usually requires the use of an operating room and incurs all of the expenses that go with that. I hate to say it, but cost seems to be a principal reason behind the continued use of the FNA. One might hope that there is some differential diagnostic process by which excisional biopsies are fast-tracked for high risk cases. From what I have learned, however, it is more often a case of cost and availability of surgeons that determines which test procedures are performed.

Email Sent December 19, 2008

This is distressing. The uncertainty is clearly the worst part. I have been flipping among three emotional states: a calm, happy, life-as-usual attitude; worst case thinking; and a dull, pervasive sense of distress. It's been a relatively long haul, with very scary as well as encouraging diagnostic results along the way -- but nothing definitive.

We have cancelled our Christmas travel plans and will now go to see our grandchildren after the operation, which is scheduled for Jan 8. The hospital system here closes the operating rooms, save to life and death emergencies, from Dec. 19 to Jan. 6! My doctor tried, in vain, to have me scheduled before the break. I find this quite frustrating, but something else I must live through.

Wait a minute! I sound depressed and morose in this email. But I was not.

My life was good. My family life was great, friends were wonderful, piano playing was plodding but enjoyable (my choir participation was on hold) and my basketball teammates were quite forgiving of my age and inadequacies. All in all, I had a pretty good life.

On January 8, I had surgery during which two procedures were completed under general anesthetic.

The surgeon removed a tumor through excisional biopsy, a more precise and complete diagnostic procedure than FNA. Definitive results were predicted for later in the week. These would determine whether the tumor was cancerous, and if so, what grade (roughly, how aggressive) and what stage (roughly, how far the cancer has progressed).

During the surgery, the doctor also performed a panendoscopy or pandoscopy, which involved inserting a flexible scope with a fibre optic camera down my throat to look for cancer in the oropharynx, the rest of the esophagus, and, I think, the trachea and bronchi (breathing tubes of the lungs). Combining this with the other scope, x-rays, ultrasounds, CT scan, five fine needle biopsies, and blood work I had had over the previous three months, we now had a very complete picture of my entire innards!

The bottom line from the pandoscopy: the specialist saw no evidence of cancer, no suspicious cells, and no reason to take additional samples for biopsy. This was a relief because all of the other tests suggested (but had not confirmed) metastatic cancer.

So, we were down to the happy conclusion that if the tumor turned out to be cancerous, it was likely removed before the cancer spread. The happier conclusion would be that the tumor was benign.

As it turned out, the surgeon was wrong.

Email Sent: January 17, 2009 – reversal of fortune

I have cancer.

That said, there is no solid information about the stage or grade of the cancer. I have now been told that the excised tumor was a secondary (metastatic) site. I do not currently understand how they know this as none of the scans and other tests have been able to locate the primary site.

14

According to the doctors, there are two "most likely" alternative ex-planations. First, the primary site is very small; it is in the head and neck area, as this is "normally the case in situations like this." Second, my immune system has already killed the primary site, so it doesn't exist anymore. If either of these assumptions is correct, then the prognosis is "very good". If these are incorrect, then the prognosis is probably bad.

The challenge would be to circumvent or at least speed up the bureaucracy. I had been told that my first appointment with a radiation specialist would happen within two weeks. That wouldn't be the start of the therapy, however, which would begin later. Frankly, this seemed too slow, especially given the amount of time I had already waited and the delays I had experienced.

Since the end of September, I had had one major surgery, five fine needle biopsies (in two sittings over two weeks), two x-rays (head and chest), two ultrasounds (neck and abdomen), CT scan (neck), two scopes put down my throat, untold blood work, and a bunch of other stuff – all punctuated by sloppy, antiquated process, bureaucratic bumbling, and a slow moving system. Now, it seemed there might be more of the same. Since there was no certainty about the location of the primary site, the search for one would be extended to include a colonoscopy, prostate biopsy (maybe), full body and head MRI, and more blood tests.

But I couldn't let this new round of diagnostics get in the way of radiation treatment!

My spirits, regardless, were still good . . .

Email Sent: January 22, 2009 – my birthday

I finally met with two oncologists today. Both are now my doctors. One is the Head of Radiation Oncology at the Ottawa Hospital. My surgical oncologist is an ENT cancer specialist. Both are very highly regarded. I am blessed to have them.

After extensive and independent examinations of me (more scopes, etc.) and my diagnostic results so far (including a few new tests I haven't written about), the doctors independently came to the same conclusions about my diagnosis and next steps.

I have squamous cell carcinoma, Stage 3, TX, N2a, MO with an as yet undetermined primary site.

Stage 3 indicates the size of the tumor; mine is 3 out of 4. Big Squamous cell carcinoma indicates relatively undifferentiated cancer cells; these are more aggressive than more differentiated cells.

TX. The "T" stands for tumor. They're not sure where the primary site is, therefore the "X" designation. No primary determined = the primary site for about 15% of head and neck cancers are never found. This does not adversely impact prognosis. N2a indicates the degree of lymph node involvement or spread (aggressiveness). Mine is diagnosed as Grade 2 (out of 4). I don't know what the "a" means.

I am being treated for head and neck cancer because, in the clinical experience of my doctors, that is what my cancer looks like. Most head and neck cancers are squamous cell carcinoma and the rest of my body appears "clean" of cancer cells.

The surgery done for excisional biopsy removed most of the tumor, but not all of it, as I found out today. This was a big surprise, as I had understood the surgeon to say that he had removed the entire tumor. My mistake, a pretty big one!

I have been admitted to a clinical trial and will have a PET (positron emission tomography) scan of my entire body to ensure that they haven't missed any cancer, and to try to find the elusive primary site.

If the PET scan shows a primary far from the neck, say in an organ like the lungs or liver, then it will be a whole new situation. If not, I will be treated for throat cancer. Once the treatment course is finished, I will have another PET scan to assess results.

Oral cancers such as mine are a mini-epidemic in Ottawa. The most probable causes are smoking and/or human papillomavirus (HPV)! HPV-16 and HPV-18 are known to cause up to 95% of cervical cancers. These two HPVs are also linked to oral cancer, the incidence of which is increasing dramatically. In part, the reason seems to be that the vagina, cervix, mouth, and throat share a similar cellular structure. No matter where it lives, HPV appears to be mutating more often. These mutations often wind up being cancerous. As the evidence for this link mounts, prominent healthcare practitioners are beginning to speak about it in public. For example, on a recent TV show, Dr. Oz and a panel of experts emphatically asked both heterosexual and homosexual North Americans to change their oral sex habits. Moreover, a federally appointed panel of experts has recently recommended the use of HPV vaccine in Canadian males.

I quit smoking 20 years ago and smoked very little for the ten years before that. But, I once was a very heavy smoker. As for sexual habits, discretion prevents any further comment.

Assuming they didn't find any metastatic sites in other parts of my body or a primary site in another part of my body, I would undergo five weeks of intense radiation of the entire neck, throat, and tongue area. This radiation therapy would entail one treatment per day for 35 days, would start within two weeks, and would "not be a picnic" as one of the oncologists put it.

By week four or five, my throat would be burned raw and very sore. I'd perhaps need a feeding tube, but if I did, it would be temporary (I'd need it for a few weeks at the most). This could be a blessed relief for those who sang with me or with whom I spoke regularly because, feeding tube or not, I wouldn't be talking much or singing near the end of the radiation treatment.

If the PET scan turned up something unexpected like a neck related primary, then I could face another, more radical surgery called a neck dissection and/or chemo. The chemo is self-explanatory. The neck dissection is the removal of all affected lymph glands and associated muscle and other tissue. At this point, neither doctor expected that the chemo would happen. The neck dissection was a different story. In many cases, the dissection is performed before the radiation therapy. I had argued against that since I hoped to avoid the surgery completely. Time would tell, of course.

Depending on how the risk factors were calculated, my odds of beating this were between 70% and 90% if there was no primary site found but as low as 56% if they did find a primary (depending on where it was). My radiation oncologist put the odds at 90% in my case. I did an independent calculation based on published risk factors to get the lower number and establish a range. He did not disagree with the range but was optimistic, at this point, about my case. Of course, the probabilities matter little; the results are what count.

Email Sent: February 8, 2009

I had a mask made for the diagnosis and treatment. That wasn't fun. The technician soaked a small piece of plastic mesh in a liquid, and then fit the mesh to me by stretching it tightly across my face. In the end, the mask is very tight fitting; it conforms to every nook and cranny of my face and neck. It has clamps on it that literally pin me to the table when I undergo diagnosis or receive each radiation treatment. I had to wear the mask for 35 minutes during the neck PET/CT scan. The experience was quite painful, and I experienced mild claustrophobia to boot. I was laid flat on the moving diagnostic bed and clamped into place. The "pillow" on the bed was made of rock hard plastic that did not contour to the shape of my head, and I could not move at all; even swallowing is not easy when clamped into place. The outline of the mesh

18

was visible on my face for 5 or 10 minutes after the test was over. It left a bunch of "mesh bubbles" on my forehead, chin, nose and cheeks.

I will wear this mask for every treatment. I'm told that the mask-wearing portion of each session will last less than 15 minutes. Nevertheless, I will probably look like a Christmas ham after every session.

Email Sent: February 9, 2009

As a result of three more CT scans and two PET scans, my diagnosis has changed somewhat. It is now Stage 4, TX, N2b, M0, squamous cell carcinoma of the ENT region. The change from Stage 3 to 4 is a bit scary, but in this type of localized ENT cancer it is much less worrisome than in other cancers, where it can be a virtual death sentence.

The N2b designation indicates that there is clear evidence of metastatic growth in three lymph nodes, all on the left side of the neck, just under the jawbone. This is a change from N2a, when they could only detect cancer in one lymph node. It turns out that my dental implants were obscuring the other affected lymph nodes. A more precise diagnostic test found these.

M0 remains the same as previously. There is no evidence of metastases in any other part of my body. This is VERY good news.

You may remember that TX = unknown primary site. Paradoxically, this is actually good in my case. In 5% of ENT squamous cell cancers, the primary is never found. The success of treatment in these cases is markedly better than in cases where they find a primary site. The reason for this is not known, but the conjecture is that the body has already killed a small primary site, which means that there is no longer a "base camp" from which cancers can be sent to colonize the body.

As for the existing metastases, squamous cells grow relatively quickly. Not likely quickly enough, though, to spread further before the treatment starts.

At the moment, my radiation therapy is set to begin sometime in the next ten days. Treatment will be once a day, Monday to Friday, for seven weeks, i.e. 35 sessions in total. There will be no chemo, and there are no plans for additional surgery. I have insisted that the docs forgo their usual protocol of surgery followed by radiation. They agreed, only after I grudgingly agreed to consider surgery if the results of the radiation were not as hoped.

The prognosis in my case has been revised to 70% to 90% chance for a complete cure. The treatment and recovery will not be pleasant, however.

The more detailed diagnosis was the result of the new tests I underwent. The PET scans (one full body and the other head and neck) were each combined with CT scans. Oversimplified, the CT scans provide a kind of map of the body upon which the PET results are overlain. The PET scan is very good at picking up cancer cells; the overlay on the CT helps pinpoint the location of the cancer. I also had a "columnar" CT of the neck that produced a number of images showing "slices" of my neck region from different angles. Taken together, the PET and the columnar CT allowed the radiologist and oncologists to "see around" the dental implants and discover the other nodal involvement (metastases).

Treatment: March / April, 2009

The treatment would be tomotherapy, five days per week for seven weeks – a total of 35 treatments. The principal advantage of tomotherapy is that it delivers radiation from 360 degrees by rotating the radiation "gun" around the patient, who is immobile on the table. It can precisely deliver radiation to a cancerous tumor using tens of thousands of tiny "beamlets" while sparing more of the normal healthy tissue around the tumor than other forms of radiation therapy. In my case, the sparing part was important because I hoped to come out of treatment with some sense of taste and some salivary function. Stray radiation, or radiation at the wrong dose, could jeopardize those happy outcomes.

On the left side of my head and neck, my radiation dosage would be the treatment maximum (70 grade) and aimed at the three affected nodes. This would completely "kill" my "left side" salivary glands (more technically, sublingual and parotid glands) and eliminate any ability for them to produce saliva.

On the right side, the dosage would be medium strength (56 grade) and aimed at the base of the tongue. It would also likely wipe out the functioning of my right sublingual salivary gland.

This approach would, however, spare my larynx and nasopharynx and my right parotid salivary gland. This was very important since it would allow me to produce some saliva after the treatment was finished.

Taken together, the certain short-term side effects of the tomotherapy form a nasty list. It includes a burning sore throat (literally a sun burnt throat) peaking in weeks four and five, maybe opiates to manage the pain in that period (this peak time is different from other radiation cases, where the worst occurs a week or two after the treatment ends); an inability to speak easily during weeks four and five; loss of taste with an uncertainty about when and whether it will return; mucous build-up in the mouth; severe dry mouth; sun burnt neck, with awful pain and peeling; possible feeding tube for a few weeks; oral fungal infections; fatigue; and loss of ability to concentrate.

Except for the feeding tube, all of these things happened. This sounds quite scary, but it became my new reality, to which I adapted quickly. I learned to live without taste and to eat by texture. I also made the transition, for a few weeks, to liquid meals. My wife cut my shirts so that they were low cut – no collars, held up only by my shoulders. This was to reduce the pain associated with touching my burnt skin. I drank carbonated water to reduce the mucous, swabbed my mouth with anti-fungals, and slept when fatigued. The one thing I did not do was wallow in my pain or feel sorry for myself. I had living to do and wellness to achieve.

In addition, I could longer sing. Unfortunately, this is a permanent side-effect, and while I do mourn the loss of my voice, I have accepted it as part of my new reality. I now play piano a lot.

Email Sent: February 12, 2009

The start of my radiation therapy has been postponed. On their third review of the PET scan, my doctors and a radiologist saw a "suspicious" area at the base of my tongue, left side. If I was not already known to have cancer, the radiologist would have called it normal. Given my condition, however, the doctors have decided to perform another biopsy to see if they have discovered the elusive primary site.

If the biopsy confirms a cancerous primary, it will be on the back third of the tongue. This part is very near the throat (pharynx). Cancers that develop here are called oropharyngeal cancers (pronounced oar-o-farin-gee-al). With ageing, oropharyngeal cancer becomes more common than all forms of oral cavity cancer except those of the lip. It is uncommon before the age of 40. The highest incidence of the disease is in males in their 60s and 70s - three times more men than women get this form of cancer. I'm 66.

The prognosis for base-of-tongue cancer with a known primary is not as good as unknown primary oral cancer. The overall cure rate is near 59%. In my case, the odds would be better, maybe in the 70% range, because the primary, if it exists, is only a small speck and I am in good shape. This is lower than an unknown primary prognosis of 80 – 90%, with the oncologists hoping for a complete cure in my case.

So, I will undergo another day surgery on February 18 to take a core sample biopsy and perhaps confirm the site visually. General anesthetic will be used but I will be home the same day. The biopsy results will be available to the oncologists on or before February 26, when I will meet with them to learn the results and hear therapy options.

No matter what the outcome of the biopsy on the 18th, we have been told that treatment will begin on March 2nd. We will know the recommendations early on February 26 and have to choose the treatment course quickly.

I'm still hopeful and relatively happy, but won't lie. This latest detour is stressful, disappointing and frustrating for Annie and me. I know the oncologists are being thorough, but I wanted to get started this week with a straightforward, high-probability-of-success therapy.

If there was no known primary, then radiation therapy would proceed as planned. Obviously, I was hoping for this because the prognosis was better than all other possible diagnoses, and the side effects would be less onerous and less long-lasting.

If I had oropharyngeal cancer with a known primary, there were four basic options:

- **Tomotherapy Radiation Alone:** To effect a cure with this method, the dosages administered to the base of my tongue would have to be dangerously high, with possible unacceptable side effects that included extreme difficulty swallowing – or never swallowing again – and having a permanent feeding tube in my stomach.

- **Tomotherapy with Brachytherapy Boost**: In my case, this method would allow a lower dose of external beam Tomotherapy to be administered to the base of my tongue, saving my ability to swallow and my right parotid salivary gland's ability to produce saliva. Brachytherapy is a radioactive "pill" that is inserted directly in the mouth as near to the primary site as possible. I'd live in a lead room for two or three days with the "pill" inside me, and visitors would be restricted to 20 minutes per visit per day. The "pill" would then be removed, and I'd go home, not radioactive. Most likely, this would be done at the end of the Tomotherapy. My radiation oncologist is one of Canada's brachytherapy experts. He treated a friend of mine with excellent results.

  Side effects would likely be as if I had unknown primary treatment: partial dry mouth, loss of taste for six months, sun burnt throat, and so on. Given the alternatives, this looked pretty appealing at the time.

- **Tomotherapy, Brachytherapy, and Neck Dissection**: This wasn't my favourite possibility. In a neck dissection procedure, lymph nodes and surrounding tissue from the neck are removed as a part of cancer treatment. The extent of tissue removal, and thus the extent of the neck dissection, varies considerably depending on the specific case. If I underwent a neck dissection, three nodes and associated tissue would be removed. It was therefore unlikely that I would undergo the most radical of dissections. Long-term side effects of neck dissections are not nice. I won't scare you with them. Unfortunately, the ENT oncologist was called to an emergency surgery during the time I was to meet him. So, I did not know what surgery might be in the offing and what damage it could do. We would find out more on the 26th if the oncologists recommend this surgery. I hoped that it was not on their treatment menu.

24

- **Tomotherapy plus Chemo:** This is a conventional treatment for oropharyngeal cancer. The choice of drug is usually dictated by the kind and stage of cancer plus the oncologists' (two in my case) comfort level with the drug. The short- and long-term toxicities associated with chemo can be quite serious, or not so bad, depending on which drug is used. A few of the specific chemo drugs favoured in my kind of oropharyngeal cancer raise the odds of bad short-term side effects, and some serious long-term toxicities.

At the time, I did not know the probabilities of cure associated with each of the above treatment regimes. I would find that out on February 26, along with the course of treatment that the oncologists recommended. Actually, they promised to present two options, with a full explanation of each.

If they *did* find a primary site, I was inclined to follow option two, with the possibility of a neck dissection after the radiation (but only if the cancer was still detectable), and I fully understood the likely long-term side effects and could live with them. I didn't know, however, if that option was included in the list of acceptable treatment protocols since neck dissections often come before radiation.

Email Sent February 19, 2009

I had the base-of-tongue biopsy/surgery on February 18. The doctor did not see any evidence of a primary site with his scope, nor did it feel like cancer when he palpated it. He took some samples – pieces of my tongue – and has sent them for biopsy.

Email Sent February 26, 2009

I met with both oncologists today. The biopsy of the base of my tongue was negative. This is good news. The doctors set the prognosis to 90%+ for a cure. As one doctor said, "You'll have dry mouth for the rest of your life, but you'll probably have to die of something else." I hope he's right.

Treatment begins next week. Radiation only; 35 treatments, once a day, 5 days/week for 7 weeks. No chemo, no plans for a neck dissection, no brachytherapy. I'll still have sore throat during treatment, no taste buds for 4-6 months and permanently lose 3 of the 4 primary salivary glands, which means I'll always have dry mouth. Funny how that doesn't sound so bad.

The oncologists and I reviewed the possible treatment regimes. They wanted to do surgery first and then radiation. I wanted to do it the other way around, hoping that the radiation would kill all of the cancer and I could avoid the surgery, which is very intrusive and potentially disfiguring. After some discussion, they agreed to treat me with radiation, and then determine if surgery was necessary.

So, my treatment began. I reported to the treatment clinic and learned the procedures I had to follow at each treatment session. At first, I found them cold, and felt like I was now part of a sausage making plant: I was the sausage, the clinic was the factory. For example, I had to swipe a bar-coded card to verify that I was in the waiting room, at which I had to appear 15 minutes before my scheduled appointment. If I didn't do either, I would lose my place in line.

The waiting room itself was large, open, and not exactly a hotbed of social activity. At any given time, the room held at least 50 people. Typically, there were a number of small groups of patients accompanied by their loved ones or caregivers. These people kept to themselves. The place was pretty quiet, not many people spoke, and when they did, it was in hushed tones. I could never figure out if this was due to their suffering, or in deference to the plight of others, or simply plain old Canadian reserve (or, perhaps, some of each). I do know that when I engaged people in conversation – and I was one of the very few who did – most people responded happily.

In stark contrast to the norm in the waiting room, when a therapist, nurse, or doctor showed up, many hitherto stone faced people would light up, smile, and march happily off to their treatment.

Over time, I came to adore the nurses, radiation therapists, nutritionists, and others who worked in that clinic. They were competent and matter-of-fact yet also positive and very hard to fluster. They interacted with people with an admirable empathy and rigor that would pass the highest tests of proficiency and kindness. If a person was upset, they understood but still did what needed to be done; if a person had trouble understanding, they helped patiently until the person got it; if a person was angry, they didn't take it personally. Almost to a person, they overwhelmed their patients with practicality and kindness. As you'll read below, this stood in sharp contrast to some of the shoddier care I received in other parts of the hospital.

As the effects of radiation began to take their toll, that cancer clinic became a very safe place for me. I trusted the healthcare workers there and looked forward to seeing them every day.

Fundraising Letter Sent March 11, 2009

I apologize for not calling first. As you know, I want to spare my voice as I go through 35 consecutive radiation treatments, which will give me a very sore throat.

As you may know, I am in a clinical trial at the Ottawa Hospital Cancer Centre. You may not know that clinical trials save lives and mine may be one of them. Clinical trials are proving grounds for treatments and adjuncts that, once validated, are then put into cancer treatment protocols. In my trial, I am undergoing PET scans to determine the exact number, size and location of metastases of my throat cancer. The PET (positron emission tomography) technique gives a very precise picture of tumors and, in my case, will allow pin point targeting of radiation doses to each of the three metastases in my neck. In other cases, drugs are tested in clinical trials; once proven these drugs can be life savers. Read on, as one is briefly described below.

I am writing to ask you to join me at a free, one hour breakfast on March 31 at the Hampton Inn to help address a crisis looming for cancer care in Ottawa. The breakfast begins at 7:15 AM and will end promptly at 8:30 AM. The breakfast is fully sponsored thanks to the generosity of the Hampton Inn and parking is free as well. We'll be in and out on time, guaranteed.

Please don't feel any pressure, but also please read on.

Here is the reason for the breakfast. The Ottawa Regional Cancer Foundation has received a special, urgent request from the Clinical Trials Office of the Ottawa Hospital Cancer Centre and the Ottawa Health Research Institute. They are at risk of closing down some trials due to funding cut-backs, which means people in Ottawa—people we care about—may not have access to all of the most innovative cancer treatment options. The doctors and researchers have asked for our help.

We will be joined by a number of oncologists and researchers, plus there will be an interesting presentation by Dr. John Bell, who heads a group of Canadian scientists developing virus based cancer therapy--viruses that kill cancer cells while leaving healthy cells untouched. This is very exciting stuff. If it proves out, in the future people in my situation will be able to avoid several very nasty and permanent side effects of conventional therapy!

Clinical trials in humans continue to be one of the fastest and safest ways for oncologists to provide better treatment options to their cancer patients and bring researchers closer to finding a cure for cancer. The Cancer Foundation is committed to continuing to fund translational research, as well as clinical trials right here in Ottawa—as there can be up to 100 on-going trials involving cancer drugs, gene therapy, trials in radiation oncology plus combinations of treatments.

The Ottawa Regional Cancer Foundation is the most significant philanthropic contributor to cancer care and research in our region. The Foundation works as a partner to improve the odds of survivorship by supporting the work being done at each of the hospitals across the region that provides cancer care.

This is a free breakfast, but it is also a fundraiser. You will be asked to make a gift, but there is no requirement to do so. The Cancer Foundation is hoping that people will give $1,000 each. But there is no minimum or maximum – people choose to give or not. Of course, tax receipts will be issued for all gifts.

If you already give, you may consider simply redirecting some of your existing gift to the clinical trials fund.

Please consider attending and joining me and my wife Anne at our table. If I am too ill from my treatments, Anne will go to the breakfast alone. She'd love company. If you cannot attend, and would like to give, we would be honoured to represent you and your gift at the event.

I look forward to hearing from you.

More than $350,000 was raised in one hour at this breakfast. I couldn't attend, but Annie did and represented us both. By the time the breakfast happened, I tired easily and was having difficulty eating and swallowing – all courtesy of the radiation treatment.

I was part of a clinical trial that was testing the efficacy of positron emission tomography (PET) as a diagnostic scanning tool. The PET scan is an alternative to MRI and CT scans. The PET procedure took the better part of three hours. First, they introduced dye into me via an IV drip and I waited for it to spread throughout my body. Once I was primed, I spent about an hour being scanned while enclosed in a very small tube. For 30 minutes my head was pinned to the table by that infernal mask. It was painful. For the next half hour, I was still in that tube while the PET device scanned my body below the neck. I didn't like undergoing the PET procedure. But, I was very grateful for the information it provided. The PET helped determine the exact location, and size of the metastatic tumors as well as how far the cancer had – and crucially – had not spread throughout my body. My treatment protocol, the targeting of the radiation, the spread of the beam and dosage had been calculated in part based on information gained in my clinical trial.

Email Sent March 20, 2009

34% of my radiation therapy is now complete. The metastatic tumors have already shrunk 50%!! Of course, as we don't know where the primary site is, we can only infer that it is also shrinking, or, as it is very small, is already eradicated. The doctor's assessment is that I am "doing very well". I'm very hopeful, and grateful for the wonderful care and support I'm receiving.

I was treated every weekday. If I was lucky, the elapsed time from the time I left until I returned was less than an hour. I had to be in the waiting room 15 minutes before the treatment was scheduled. If the machine was down and needed re-calibrating or if there was an emergency, I could be away from home for two hours or more. One day per week, I saw my radiation oncologist and a dietician, which added another hour to the process.

I had walked to many appointments and driven to others. The actual treatment time was 20 minutes, all in that uncomfortable mask. The tomotherapy radiation was delivered for eight of those minutes; the rest of the time involved a combination of positioning me for the treatment and a CT scan to ensure targeting accuracy. This scan also measured the size of the tumors. The therapists (two each time) were all very competent. As one would expect, however, some were kinder and more personable than others.

Over time, I had made my peace with the mask. It was still uncomfortable, hellishly so some days, but bearable. I meditated for the entire therapy session. This helped me deal with the mask and forget the noise in the room. The machine was noisy to begin with, and doubly so when delivering the radiation (remember, the radiation is delivered from various spots in a 360 degree arc). It was a rattling sound with a boring beat that traveled around my head.

There was always a specialist nurse available to deal with things like pain management (e.g., sore throat) and other issues (e.g., thrush and mucus build-up). Because pain medication becomes less effective with use, I had refrained from taking any at this point; I wanted the drug's effectiveness to be optimal when I really need it. I also wanted to avoid serious opiates if I could.

The following week, I would have my mask re-evaluated to see if it still fit properly. If not (e.g., if I had lost too much weight), then they would make another, tighter one. Oh, joy! Fortunately, I was only down a pound or two.

Email Sent April 4, 2009

I have now finished 22 of 35 treatments. Due to Easter break and weekends, the radiation therapy will last until April 24.

Side effects are peaking and most, but not all, will likely now plateau until the end of therapy. They will begin to dissipate within three weeks, with rapid improvement expected a week or so after they begin to disappear.

The insides of my mouth and throat are already burnt and scabbed. I am tender where I am supposed to be tender, my throat is constricting (I drink purées rather than eating), my mouth is always dry. Mucus is thick without saliva, so I am constantly drinking carbonated water (breaks up the mucus). From now on, my mouth will always be dry, but I should get minimal salivary function back relatively fast once the treatments end. I am also being treated for thrush, a fungal infection that can be quite painful. They don't treat this in advance, only if it shows up, using anti-fungal medication. Approximately 75% of ENT radiation patients get it. No big deal; it will end when the treatments end.

The skin on my neck was beginning to burn. Although it looked and felt like a sunburn, it was a slightly different phenomenon. I treated it first with Aloe Vera, later with more serious creams, all of which I had to pat on, not rub on. This was a side effect that would keep getting worse until the end of radiation.

I also had a bear of a bladder infection that kept me from sleeping for a week or so. The doctor prescribed antibiotics which kicked in and sweet sleep finally returned.

The most surprising thing was taste. As expected, mine was virtually gone. Everything tasted vaguely metallic; this was caused by the blood constantly dripping down my throat. I had some taste left, but the risk remained that it, too, would go completely. I couldn't distinguish many flavours. When I did detect a flavour, it was difficult to enjoy as it was always accompanied by that underlying metallic "taste".

I could only tolerate certain foods – acidic foods like fruit and foods that require a lot of chewing were off the menu. The list of foods I could eat was fairly uninspiring, high in protein, soft and bland, very close to puréed. Swallowing was difficult. The inside of my throat was swelling and constricting. I had to crush pills to get them down, for example, and eat soft foods.

My throat was constantly sore. This was expected to get worse before it got better. All of that notwithstanding, I actually learned to "like" certain foods. I ate by texture, not taste. As this sensibility developed, it produced some surprises. For example, I hated ice cream. To me it "tasted" like cold toothpaste, not the soothing, smooth balm for the throat one might expect.

When I first read that my taste buds would be eradicated, I assumed that the effect would only manifest itself when I ate or drank something. Not true: 24/7 my mouth tasted of metal with a soup-con of salt (delightful) whether or not I was eating or drinking. I tasted nothing else, and only sensed textures. My taste buds would take at least three to six months to return. The prediction was that my sense of taste would come back in stages; probably not 100%, closer to 60%. The reality is that it is still at about 40%, some two and half years after treatment.

I was tired and losing weight. The radiation-induced fatigue could be brutal, sometimes so pervasive that I had to will myself to think. As treatment progressed, that crushing fatigue began to wane. Weariness would probably last a bit longer than the other side effects, but it would no longer be debilitating. Because I was in good shape at the time, I didn't expect fatigue to be a problem for long. I was, in fact, holding low energy somewhat at bay with regular, almost daily, exercise (long, brisk walks and some weights).

At one point, my metabolic rate doubled. I had to pour calories into me at an alarming rate. I ate copious quantities of mush five or six times a day, and even drank a can of Ensure once or twice a day. I was fighting the reverse battle of the bulge. Eating was not pleasant: even the best textures hurt on the way down, and I did not like force feeding myself to keep my weight up. Despite my best efforts, I was barely holding my own. I had lost eight or nine pounds since the beginning of the process. Although I did not like it, my wife's insistence on sticking to the force feeding regime paid off. My weight stabilized. The high calorie but still healthy mush did its job.

I had dry mouth and mucus build-up. It felt at the time like almost all of my saliva was gone. I used soda water (carbonation plus baking soda), which helped to replace the hygiene usually supplied by saliva and to break up naturally occurring mucus, which becomes thick and ropey without the saliva to dilute it. I also drank a lot of sparkling water, which also helped with mucus and partially alleviated the dry feeling. My saliva has not come back.

Despite these truly horrible side effects, I stayed focused on getting better and living life as fully as I could. I wrote, went for walks, read, tried to play the piano, tried to work a bit and, to some extent, visited with people.

So far, I'd been receiving radiation therapy only. Was the treatment effective? Every clinical indicator was positive. For example, the tumors began shrinking; the radiation was hitting the targets in the intended dosages. After each weekly exam, the doctor was more optimistic that the therapy was working. He was quite conservative, a one-step-at-a-time kind of guy. He was, however, still holding out a 60% chance that I would have a modified radical neck dissection eight weeks after the end of radiation. This was surprising since he had earlier put the probability for the neck dissection much lower.

Why the reversal? The clinical protocol I was participating in studied the predictive, diagnostic accuracy of PET scans. Apparently, the evidence coming in from this study, and others, was undermining the doctor's willingness to rely on PET scan results. So, even if the post-treatment PET and columnar CT scans were negative, they could still urge the dissection just to be sure that they had eliminated all of the cancer. Of course, I was not happy about this. Modified or not, radical neck dissections are not pleasant. Who wants to have half of his or her neck removed?

Email Sent May 7, 2009 – decision to do neck dissection

I am going to have a modified radical neck dissection. Frankly, this is the scariest decision I have made about my cancer therapy. Here's why. The surgeon will dissect and remove most of the left side of my neck. This includes lymph glands, other glands, muscle; it may also entail cutting one or more nerves to my face and shoulder. In a worse case, the dissection may entail removing some of my jaw, although this is not likely. What happens during surgery will depend on what the surgeon sees. If he sees something suspicious, he'll cut it out.

Why did Annie and I decide on surgery? After my radiation therapy was finished, I had an MRI and CT scan. The idea was to determine if any cancer cells were left. The results were ambiguous, dammit. There is a small shadow on the scan. It could be cancer, it could be something else. If it is a remnant of cancer, the cells could be in their death throes, or they could be thriving. There is no way to tell.

My radiation oncologist put the choice to me in simple terms. He said, "Look, except for this one question, we've treated you successfully. Although the odds are that this is not cancer, we don't know for sure . . . and, I've seen things like this turn out to be malignancies. Your chances of survival are very high if you have the surgery now. We aren't very successful treating cancers of this type later on if they keep spreading.

My wife simply looked at me. Her eyes spoke volumes. I couldn't bear the thought of putting her through another ordeal of caring for an invalid, especially one who was too stubborn to make a simple decision in favour of surgery.

I had already had a very debilitating course of radiation therapy. Surgery was the next step. The surgeon's Fellow, one step beyond a Resident, called it "the suspenders and belt approach." Made sense to me, I wouldn't want to get caught with my pants down on this one. I did not relish another round of treatment, this time entailing poisonous chemical cocktails and certain surgery, not to mention more radiation if the cancer spread to another part of my body.

So, I decided to have the surgery.

About two weeks after the end of the radiation treatments, my wife and I prepared and planted a garden. It was a beautiful spring, so I literally dug in. I became stronger every day. We built some enclosures to keep creatures out of the gardens, prepared raised beds and planted a slew of vegetables. To help protect my neck from the sun, I worked only in the early morning or late afternoon. Even then, I wrapped my neck with UV resistant scarves, wore a big floppy UV resistant hat and almost bathed in sun screen.

Planting that garden was a simple, satisfying pleasure. The irony of it was not lost on me, however. As a young man, I had been inspired by a (probably apocryphal) story about St. Francis of Assisi. As the story goes, St. Francis was hoeing his garden. He was asked what he would do if he knew he was going to die a horrible death in two hours. He said that he would finish the garden.

The prospect of surgery scared me more than anything else in my cancer journey. A radical neck dissection (modified or not) can result in disfigurement, including bad scarring, permanently distorted facial features, partial paralysis of the face and the removal of a jawbone. Another common side effect is a dropped and /or frozen shoulder, where one shoulder is permanently lower than the other, strength on that side of the body is severely reduced, movement is compromised, and the shoulder blade sticks out.

The surgeon didn't sugar coat these possibilities. In keeping with my insistence on being an informed patient, we discussed them openly and in detail.

I struggled with these horrid prospects while doing the garden – and reflecting more than once about St. Francis. By the time the date for my surgery arrived, I had dealt with my fears, but remained nervous – wondering which if any of the side effects I would have.

Of course I felt emotions, but I was not pre-occupied with

them. I am not unique in this – many of the cancer survivors I have coached have been the same. In my opinion, it is not good therapy to indulge in emotionalism – better to acknowledge your fears, angers and positive emotions and turn that energy to helping the healing process.

Surgery: June 19, 2009

Check-in at the hospital on the day of surgery is a crap shoot. A nurse usually does the intake, asking questions, taking BP and other vitals, etc. In my experience, and I have undergone a number of surgeries, the quality of the intake varies considerably. Some nurses are excellent, while others seem to have slept through their training. Unfortunately, for every good admitting nurse, I have had three bad ones. I won't go into too much detail, but the problems seem to be related to attitude (poor to bored), poor procedures for taking vital signs (in particular BP), and/or inability to take clear notes – even with a step-by-step checklist in hand.

Here are some examples: during admission on the day of my modified radical neck dissection, a nice and cheery nurse asked how much I weighed. I told her that I wasn't sure, that I had varied by ten pounds over the last week, and I gave her the range: 162 to 172. She said: "Oh that's OK, all we need is an estimate." She never weighed me! Did she not know that anesthetic doses are measured in milligrams per kilogram of body weight? I corrected this problem with the anesthesiologist before surgery.

Same woman, later in the admission interview . . .

Nurse: "Do you have any dental work?"

Me: "Yes, I have caps in the upper front and five implants in the lower jaw, three on the left, two on the right."

Nurse: "Have you ever had hepatitis?"

Me: "Yes"

Nurse: "What kind?"

Me: "It was called Hepatitis X, caused by an allergy to clavulinic acid."

Nurse: "What's that? I've never heard of it. Do you have any implants?"

She also insisted, twice, that I was having a "ratified radical neck dissection" as she read from forms that clearly stated "modified radical neck dissection." When I corrected her, she corrected me.

Before a different surgery, a nurse coughed and sneezed her way into the room without a face mask, handling instruments that would be used on me, started to take my BP before I had even sat down and while asking me questions to which she expected immediate replies (all procedural no-nos). I asked her why she had come to work and exposed people undergoing and recovering from surgery to her flu, and she said, "I had to. I need the money, and if I didn't come, we'd be short staffed." I asked her why she was violating procedure, and she said that she was in a hurry.

On the other hand, the care in the operating and recovery rooms are mostly excellent. In my case, I was interviewed by a nurse, an anesthesiologist, and the surgeon before the operation. All went through a checklist of questions, even to the point of indicating the point of the incision on my skin with a marker. Each person was intelligent in his or her questioning and explored the implications of my answers. In other words, they didn't dumbly follow the checklist.

This care and intelligent attention to detail continued in the operating room. While the operating room people and procedures were superb, the surgery itself was brutal.

When you are asleep during an operation, you breathe through an intubation tube. Usually, people are intubated after they have been anesthetized. Instead, to mitigate risks caused by my radiation therapy, I underwent a technique called an awake intubation. During this procedure, the anesthesiologist froze my throat with a local anesthetic, threaded a camera through the intubation tube, put the camera down my throat, and used its images to guide the tube into place. After the tube was properly inserted, they pulled the camera out through it and put me to sleep. In order to reduce the unpleasant memories associated with the awake intubation procedure, they administered drugs that produce retrograde amnesia. In my case, these drugs seemed to make me ill after the surgery, but didn't erase all of the memories. So, I was able to experience and remember lots of stuff that happens in the operating room after patients are usually asleep: positioning of the body, some pretty frank and unvarnished conversations, and so on.

Email Sent June 23, 2009

The surgery went very well. My surgeon, did all that he needed to do in a little over three hours, instead of the four he had estimated. There were no glitches or complications. He saw no evidence of cancer. As we had agreed before the surgery, he took a conservative approach by exploring the left side of my neck widely and sacrificing a lot of lymph nodes – potential metastatic sites in which microscopic cancer might be hiding. I want to eliminate all of the cancer, even the microscopic stuff that can't yet be seen. At the same time, he agreed to spare what nerves, muscle tissue and glands as he could. And he did just that, only dissecting 4 of the 5 zones in the neck.

My surgeon called the operation a success from all points of view. My medical friends, two of whom have worked in the cancer thoracic surgery unit (my temporary home for the brief hospital stay), have marveled at the surgeon's work – the "artful" incision, the "clean" healing and how good things look for recovery.

I am very hopeful. The doctor told my wife that he saw no evidence of active cancer, nor "is there any reason for suspicion." Nevertheless, he sent a number of tissue samples for biopsy. We will know the results in two weeks. He told me that, although he can't be sure, he does not expect to find any cancer. Obviously, I hope that he is right.

Aside from people in the operating room and post-surgical recovery, care from the support staff at the hospital was generally adequate to poor. Some glaring examples of poor care are given above, more follow below. These problems seem to be best explained by overcrowding, sliding standards, cost cutting, counter intuitive contractual terms for doctors and nurses, and mindless adherence to generalized guidelines and protocols. That said, however, poor training and sloppy attitudes also seem to play a large part.

Hospital Ward Vignette 1:

I pushed the "call" button during my first and only morning in the hospital after surgery.

Voice from a speaker: "Can I help you 15-2?" (Although groggy, I quickly figured out that that was me, room 6115, bed 2).

Me: "I am very nauseous. I have nothing to throw up into; I only have a drinking cup."

Voice: "We'll be right there."

12 minutes later by the clock in front of my bed, I pushed the "call" button again.

Same voice: "Can I help you 15-2?"

Me: "You may remember that I called earlier. I am vomiting now . . . I have tubes in me, a large incision in my neck and my cup will soon runneth over, if you know what I mean."

Voice: "Jane, go to 15-2 stat."

Jane came in quite quickly and gave me a container into which to vomit. As soon as she spoke to me, I recognized Jane as the voice who for the previous twelve minutes had been discussing vacation plans with a friend just outside my door.

Hospital Ward Vignette 2:

About sixteen hours after surgery, the drainage tube in my neck stopped working. I had been told that the tube would be in my neck for two to three days and that I would probably be in hospital for that time. When the tube stopped draining, a young doctor was called to look at it.

She: "Looks like there is nothing more to drain. I'll remove it."

Me: "I'm very drowsy but that doesn't sound right. I don't think you should remove the tube yet. Where's my doctor?"

She: "He's not here. Don't you want to go home? If I take this tube out, you can go home."

Me: "Who wouldn't want to go home (from care like this)?"

She: "Good, I'll take it out."

Me: "No. It's probably only clogged by a blood clot. Use an anti-coagulant."

She: "Too late."

Me: "Let me see that. Looks like a blood clot to me."

I left the hospital in a post-anesthetic fog, my face still orange from the operating room, and looking like someone had blown up a balloon in the left side of my head. In a clear violation of hospital policy, I did not even have the benefit of a wheelchair or person to accompany us to the front door. Nurse Jane apologized and said,

"I'm sorry, but we're very short-staffed as this is a holiday (Father's Day) weekend. You'll probably find a chair along the way." We didn't. It was a long walk; Annie literally held me up for most of it. The wait at the door while Annie retrieved the car was tiring and a bit scary. I was disoriented and in danger of losing consciousness.

Everything I've read and been told says that I should have stayed in hospital for another day or two. Staff at the hospital apologized quietly and quickly changed the subject. I didn't push the matter because I didn't want to piss off the people who were still going to care for me.

That said, we had two very frightening days at home. It was a holiday weekend, so apart from an overcrowded and understaffed emergency room, it was difficult to see medical people. Besides, I was too weak and drugged to move easily and I didn't want to spend hours in a germ infested emergency room. So we waited for the excess fluid and cellular matter that should have been draining to be absorbed internally. I was so swollen that Annie was afraid that my airway might be blocked if I slept in the wrong position. Two friends who are former thoracic cancer nurses confirmed that this was a valid concern. Annie got very little sleep as she watched me to make sure that I was breathing while I was asleep.

During these two days, I was taking a prescribed painkiller. I had told the hospital staff that opiates and I do not get along. They assured me that the pills I was to take were safe for me. It turns out that they contained an opiate, and they produced a rather horrific set of delusions and perceptual distortions. At one point, I firmly believed that Annie and our nurse friend were plotting to kill me. They had washed the blood off of the surgical staples in my neck that were used to hold the wound closed. I believed that I could see the staples rusting, that this was making them constrict and would choke me, and that the rust was going to cause an infection. How convenient, I thought. The perfect crime. I would die from surgical complications and no one would be the wiser. The drug wore off; I didn't take any more, and the crazy thinking stopped.

First stages of recovery: June to August, 2009

Email Sent June 25, 2009

My surgery on June 19 took just over three hours. As you know, they sent me home from the hospital less than 24 hours after the operation was completed. I arrived home confused, weak, swollen and in some pain. I think the confusion was an after effect of the anesthetic – this was my third general in less than six months – and the opiate based painkiller I took for a day.

All in all, my modified radical neck dissection was not a pleasant experience. Recovery from the operation has been difficult. I've had a tough time. Fatigue, soreness and other post-operative effects have made day-to-day living and working a chore (yes, I have had to work, albeit part-time, through this). Some people have been very understanding about the challenges I face, while others have been remarkably insensitive. This surprised me for about a nanosecond. Then, I remembered that it is part of the human condition.

The recovery process is slowly getting easier.

Email Sent June 30, 2009

All of the staples in my neck were removed today. This is a tremendous relief. Their purpose was to hold the incision together, to help it heal. On discharge from hospital, there were at least 36 staples in my neck and throat, arranged in a flattened "Y" shape. The top part of this zipper-like figure runs from behind my left ear to the midline of my throat about where the neck meets the skin under the jaw. The straight part of the "Y" is slightly curved, and runs down from under the midline of my jaw to the clavicle. My face and neck were like a lopsided balloon, grotesquely swollen in some places and stapled taut in others. By day four, the staples were very uncomfortable, making it difficult to sleep – or even move my head in certain ways.

I could have easily passed for one of Frankenstein's ugly cousins. If it walks like a duck, talks like a duck, moves like a duck . . . As a good friend said: "36 is one hell of a lot of staples in one neck -- but then maybe it allows you to remove your head at bedtime and leave it on the bedside table."

The doctor pronounced that I was in good shape, said the swelling would come down gradually over the next six months, and indicated that I may have some fluid retention in my neck for that long as well.

Smiling and speaking? I had a bit of difficulty with the lower lip, left side. It improved over the following few days, but I still had a lopsided smile, a minor speech impediment, and drooped lip. It looked not unlike the effects of a minor stroke, but was in fact a case of nerve fatigue; likely, I had some peristhesia too since there was numbness and tingling. Some parts of my jaw were completely numb, while other parts felt much like a dentist's anesthetic wearing off. I hoped that the nerve would work well again someday, but there were no promises. Pushed for a probability, the surgeon gave a 60% chance of a full recovery but higher likelihood of significant improvement.

There were no apparent long term problems with the left shoulder. I had full movement, no droopiness, but some pain that was sporadic yet diminishing progressively (likely associated with the angle of my arm and shoulder during surgery). I could play the piano as poorly as ever, but couldn't, at that point, use my left arm effectively on the basketball court. I was now cleared to begin to build up my strength and stamina slowly, so I got on with that. It wouldn't be a problem because I love a number of sports and hiking in the country.

Email Sent: July 21, 2009

Annie and I met with the surgical oncologists on July 16 for a post-operative consultation and evaluation. It turns out that there were two surgeons. As one said, "You can't really do this kind of surgery alone."

We were mainly interested in the results of the biopsy of the tissue samples that had been removed from my neck during surgery. They knew from previous images exactly where the metastatic tumors had been and were hoping the surgery would answer a few key questions:

Were the tumors gone? Was there any sign of cancer anywhere else? If so, how far had it migrated from the known sites? And so on.

Both surgeons seem quite convinced that the operation was a total success. Neither of them saw any sign of cancer, both said the operation went perfectly and saw indications that I had "responded extremely well to radiation therapy." Neither surgeon expects a negative biopsy report.

That said, the main result of the meeting was that, as of July 21, there were no biopsy results. There was no technical reason for this. Instead, it seems that sloppy succession planning was the culprit. A pathologist had retired, and there was no one to take his or her place, so there was a "backlog." The frustrating thing was that much of the technical work to get the biopsy results was already done. The tissue processing was complete; histology (thin slices of tissue) and smears had been prepared by technicians. We were simply awaiting the availability of an expert to read them.

We did not know when we would get the biopsy results. The surgeons were going on vacation for two weeks and their office was closing during that time! One actually said, "Hopefully, your results will be ready next week when you meet your other oncologist; otherwise, you'll find out after we get back because he's on vacation after next week, too." So, we would find out July 23 when we met my head oncologist or else sometime in August.

Think about this for a minute. Ever wonder how it feels to be part of a backlog when your life could be a stake?

This was simply one more unconscionable delay in a series of systemic missteps that occurred throughout my cancer journey. Each mistake resulted in a delay, lost result, etc. When added together, these probably mean that my cancer grew a lot during the prolonged diagnostic process and was more difficult to treat as a result.

My worry, however, was small compared to others. The chances that I still had cancer were by then quite low. Early in my cancer journey, I had experienced delayed and inappropriate testing as well. During these delays my cancer went from Stage two to Stage four, and the metastatic spread of the cancer probably increased. Yet I was lucky. Others, some of whom I know, have experienced similar problems getting tests and results and are now dead or dying. One wonders if that need be the case or whether their deaths are at least partially induced by the system that is charged with curing them. It is worth noting that errors of omission and commission in medical testing in Ontario, Alberta, B.C., Saskatchewan, and Newfoundland and Labrador have all been in the press in the past few years, causing those provinces to order reviews and corrective actions.

The next time you hear the political catch phrase "reducing waiting times," please think about how these remedies need to be thought through and carefully targeted in order to eliminate the human tragedies involved.

Email Sent July 23, 2009

My oncologist received the biopsy report just moments before our appointment today. He read it for the first time with Annie and me. The news is good. I appear to be cancer free.

The report shows that the pathologist examined 30 lymph nodes that had been removed from zones 1 to 4 in my neck. There were two important findings:

28 nodes were negative for cancer; 2 were positive. The nodes that contained cancer cells were in zone 2 of my neck, the location of the largest, and first, metastatic tumor; probably left over from it. The cancer cells only showed up after staining, and were quite small. They might or might not have been in the last stage of cell necrosis (death) as a result of the radiation. In any case, they are gone now.

There was no evidence of "extra" nodal cancer or further meta-static spread of the disease. The only cancer they found was the remnants of my first tumor.

Although the doctor repeated that the probability for a complete cure remains very high, he will follow me for three years before declaring it a fact. My next appointment is at the end of September, and I will be scanned again in October/November.

The doctor told me to go and live the rest of my life.

Part Two

Reflections and Observations

It is now two and half years since my radiation treatment. I have had time to reflect a bit on what having cancer has meant to me and to recall some events that made an impression on me.

Conversation During Diagnosis

I wrote this right after a particularly vexing interaction with a doctor's office. It was during the height of the uncertainty about my diagnosis,

My question: "Will you call and tell me the results when they come in?"

Answer: "No. It's against policy. If we did this for you, we'd have to do it for everyone. We'll call and set up an appointment."

Me: "Wait a minute. I am everyone. This is a universal health-care system; isn't it supposed to care for me and everyone else the same?"

Answer: "We don't have time to call everyone."

Me: "But you have time to call to book an appointment?"

Answer: "My secretary does that. We like to tell you the results in person. I always want to see a person to deliver bad news, so if I gave good news on the phone and bad during appointments, people

would get to know that an appointment means bad news. This could create unnecessary anxiety."

Me: *"But your secretary told me that if there was bad news, you would call and schedule an appointment urgently; you'd fit me in. So, I'd know there was bad news anyway, just not the details. Since you are telling me that I need an appointment to get my results, if I were prone to anxiety I would now become anxious trying to figure out whether the date of the appointment indicated a sense of urgency. Besides, other doctors have called me with cancer results, positive and negative. Those calls took less time than an appointment. With the bad news, my fears were allayed effectively and an appointment, usually for a test followed by a consult, was booked quickly. The whole process was sped up and more efficient than had I gone through the extra step of a consult before the test."*

And so on. Am I sounding anxious yet?

I can't help wondering how much of this "policy" is rooted in the billing opportunity an appointment offers, and how much it is rooted in some bureaucratic process, a misdirected cost-effectiveness measure, or a contractual restriction imposed by the billing system for doctors. It certainly is hard to see how the patient's concerns and well being come first in all of this.

Please don't misunderstand. I am not painting the health care system and people who work in it as all bad. You already know from my emails how much I admire certain people and am grateful to them and for the tools the system provides. I do mean, however, to hold a mirror up to even the good people when what they do needs tweaking or even an overhaul.

Lessons from the Radiation Treatment Centre

The radiation treatment centre is a strange mixture of comprehensive treatment, efficiency, warmth, humour, fear, suffering, anger, and hope. At some level, every patient, and probably every professional, is acutely aware that his or her birth certificate has an expiration date. Some may even have a good idea what that date is.

I spent nearly an hour in the treatment centre four days a week and nearly two and half hours one other day per week. In that time, I came to see how different people react to the threat of cancer in different ways and how reactions can change as treatment progresses.

Cancer Is an Equal Opportunity Disease

Cancer does not appear to respect lifestyles. You can contract cancer no matter what you eat, how you exercise, how much stress you have in your life, how many vitamins you take, how much you meditate, and so on. In the treatment centre, I've seen athletes, smokers, health nuts, plain nuts, heavy drinkers, non-drinkers, old people, children, rich people, poor people, and just plain ordinary folk. Cancer's etiology seems to be a hodge-podge of genetics, environment, and lifestyle habits. If, for example, you have the wrong genes, then it'll get you.

There was a famous Tai Chi teacher and doctor in Ottawa who lived an exemplary life of kindness and service. He was known for his joy and for his disciplined approach to diet and exercise. He died of cancer at the age of 56! All of the males in his family had died of the same cancer at the age of about 45. Did his lifestyle give him an extra decade? Who knows? Did it protect him from cancer? No.

There was a little boy whose dad pushed him around the cancer centre in a wheel chair. The boy was bald and weak, yet he played happily with his toys and laughed easily. He had an almost stoic acceptance of his lot. Every staff member who treated him lit up in his presence. I think he died during the fourth week of my treatment.

A busy executive came in for his first treatment, Blackberry blazing. He strode back and forth, speaking to people on the phone, sending emails, and looking at his watch. It was as if he had a meeting to get to and didn't want the treatment (for prostate cancer) to make him late. He wasn't rude to anyone, but clearly didn't look like he wanted to speak with anyone, including the staff. Three weeks later, he was a different person: slower, kinder to people around him, grateful for staff help. He is now in remission.

Sometimes, when waiting for my weekly appointment with the doctor or the dietician, I would sit in another part of the centre, the place where chemo is given. Staff would administer the chemo to people lying in beds across from the waiting room chairs. These patients varied from people reading books to living cadavers.

Another guy came to every treatment with his two sons. He had throat cancer and usually became so nervous waiting for his treatment that he and one of his sons would go out for a smoke; sometimes he appeared as if he'd been drinking as well. He did this for the three weeks I observed him. He reminded me of the grossly overweight guy who had by-pass surgery in the same week I had mine. At our "graduation" seminar, he listened politely and then announced that all of this after care stuff was good to know, but he was going to go out and have a smoke and a few good drinks.

These last two are extreme examples. There are, however, a lot of people who are cut of the same cloth. They wear it more conservatively but undermine their treatment or post-treatment recovery nevertheless because they don't make the necessary adjustments to take care of themselves.

I can't help wondering what to do with people like that, people who ignore easily accessible information about diet, exercise, and lifestyle choices that are known to help with treatment and recovery. It's not that they aren't exposed to the facts in the cancer clinics. In my experience, the system bends over backwards to give people access to nutritional advice, fitness assessments, supervised exercise regimes, counseling, physiotherapy, and so on. There are so many people who try hard to make changes to their lifestyles during and after treatment. Why should they be treated the same as people who don't and who take up valuable places in a backlogged system, the capacity of which is stressed and stretched? I know my wondering sounds almost heretical, but shouldn't people be responsible for meeting minimal lifestyle milestones, especially after diagnosis, in order to receive equal priority in the system? By the same token, perhaps the system should make greater efforts to encourage opportunities for the patient to partner with the healthcare providers on lifestyle issues.

This is not merely my question; it is a genuine ethical issue for the healthcare system. In some cases, people are required to make lifestyle changes to receive medical treatment. For example, a man I know was refused a kidney transplant until he lost 25 pounds, even though his kidney function was low enough to warrant immediate action.

Focused Acts of Kindness

The patient load at the treatment centre (and all others in Canada) is immense, and cancer rate is increasing. It seems to be the disease of our age. Statistics are scary; one reputable source has said that soon one in three people in Canada will be touched by cancer!

The treatment centre is business-like. It has to be. For example, each patient gets an appointment card with a bar code on it. When I arrived for each appointment, I had to swipe the code over a scanner. That told the system that I was there and ready for treatment. My doctor once said about the efficiency of the place, "If you snooze, you lose." If I didn't swipe the code, I'd miss my place in the treatment line.

Yes. That's only one example; the centre is business-like in many ways. Therapies are delivered efficiently, doctors and nurses don't waste time, systems and processes are clock-work smooth. But, there was something else, something equally important in the way doctors, nurses, therapists, clerks, and other healthcare providers dealt with patients.

Almost to a person, they were smart and kind. I can't tell you enough how important kindness is in that setting. Patients can be anxious, confused, angry, helpless, scared. Sometimes, all at once! Rarely does a cancer treatment worker meet a patient at his or her best, or even close to it.

After dealing with so many people who were "just doing my job" during the diagnosis, I was happily surprised to find professionals with years of clinical experience who care and who show it. In my case, they discerned that I needed to deal with my cancer factually, empirically, and with a sense of humour. I couldn't stand sanctimonious, paternalistic care. No one soft peddled problems or tried to bullshit me. Once they got to know me, they dealt with me straight up. I felt like a partner in the treatment process. They were willing to discuss technical details with me; they made sure that Annie and I both could see the monitors as they put scopes down my throat and described the results in real time; we looked at the PET and CT results with them, and so on. They neither belittled nor pandered to my research findings and questions. They didn't flaunt their knowledge but discussed treatment options with me. They didn't try to infantilize me but listened to and weighed what I said. I felt safe with this team. I needed that.

Most of the other patients I spoke with passively accepted their treatment, didn't know much about it, and didn't want to. They seemed content with the basics: showing up when they were told to, taking medicine as directed, and the like.

In another sense, they were a varied lot. Some were demanding (I want my treatment now!), some were emotionally overwrought, some started out angry, some were emotionless, some were curious, some were bewildered, some were so sick they really didn't care, some didn't seem to understand even the basics, and others just wanted to know what to do next. Despite these marked differences in perspective and personality, everyone told me how happy he or she was with the treatment experience, how kind and capable the providers were. The treatment staff did a remarkable job dealing with patients in a way that made them comfortable yet got the job done. This speaks volumes for the skills and kindness of the staff.

I remember being inspired by Anne Herbert in the late 70s and early 80s, who wrote "practice random acts of kindness and senseless acts of beauty" on place mats and left them in a restaurant in Sausalito, California. It seemed such a simple and necessary idea to me. Apparently, I wasn't the only one. People noticed, and it has now turned into a movement of sorts. It still needs more adherents and daily practitioners…throughout the healthcare system, and throughout society.

Education and Myth Busting

At the treatment centre, I learned that people need to take responsibility for their health and medical care. Doctors and nurses need our help. It doesn't do them or us as patients any good to mythologize their abilities, to put them on pedestals. They are busy; they can and do overlook things or make mistakes. We need to inform ourselves about cancer, about its treatment and to take responsibility for our part in its prevention and cure. We need to be active partners in our cure, not passive pieces of meat in the cancer treatment process.

That said, some doctors and healthcare workers hide behind arrogance, perhaps because it helps distance themselves from patients, perhaps because they are full of themselves. Who knows? What I do know is that arrogance must be met with kindness and a dogged insistence that treatment is a partnership between health-care providers and the patient. Both have responsibilities and ac-countabilities in the process. Patients, for example, have a responsibility to be informed and engaged, not childlike and pass-ive. They also have a responsibility to engage their doctors and other providers in meaningful relationships, to ask questions, to look for options and evaluate them.

As I came to know my dietician, she remarked that I was an unusual patient. Why? Because I knew my body, knew enough about nutrition and exercise to help her do her job, and was willing to follow appropriate diet and exercise regimens without com-promise. One of her jobs is to obsess about weight loss during a person's cancer treatment. She found it remarkable that I didn't lose much weight (relatively speaking), and was already taking steps to make sure it would stay that way.

As I had a heart-related need to eat as low a cholesterol diet as possible, yet not lose weight, this proved challenging. She was happy to give practical advice tailored to my rather unique situ-ation. She also told me that my weight loss numbers were in the top four or five of her patients.

The same pattern repeated itself with the rest of the treatment team and their regime. We acquired enough critical and detailed knowledge about radiation therapy, surgery, exercise, diet and nu-trition, and the entire gamut of the treatment process to contribute meaningfully to treatment discussions and to cause positive out-comes in the treatment by our behaviour and habits. Ultimately, the doctors and others came to respect and encourage this. We worked out a relationship that respected their authority and knowledge, while encouraging discussion and mutual weighing of treatment options.

We even made minor contributions. For example, the skin on my neck and collarbone burnt very badly during the radiation, so much so that Annie cut the necks off of a number of my shirts. Even so, it was painful to wear a shirt, and very difficult to sleep. The nurses had recommended a number of creams for the burns and one in particular. It helped, but not as much as another cream I found through my pharmacist. This cream was new and not widely known but had been used successfully in a cancer treatment trial out west. The nurses followed my course of treatment with the new cream and wound up recommending it to others.

At every turn, healthcare providers welcomed our insistence on being responsible, knowledgeable partners in my care. My oncologist remarked that my chances of recovery were enhanced by my attitude, the support network we built and the emphasis I put on being an active participant and informed, realistic decision maker as a patient. So, my question is this: why was my behaviour as a patient so different that many of those who cared for me commented on it? Why aren't there more people who actively immerse themselves in their treatment? After all, when you have a serious disease, it is your most important job.

My answer is this. Many people either don't know how to advocate for their own care in a responsible and knowledgeable way or else they choose not to do so. For some, it boils down to not knowing how to have a sustained "adult conversation" with their healthcare providers and with doctors in particular. For example, I've seen otherwise accomplished people behave like infants with their doctors and nurses. They become passive recipients of diagnostic procedures and treatments ("Whatever you say, doctor"). Maybe they are intimidated; maybe they are socialized to be in awe of doctors and healthcare providers, to see them as all-knowing. Whatever the reason, they don't inform themselves or penetrate the cloud of medical jargon. To be a responsible patient, one needs to learn some medical terms and, more important, medical concepts.

I've witnessed others, a much smaller group, who are wary of traditional health care providers, who see them almost as necessary evils or who restrict themselves to alternative medicine. In my view, these people miss the boat, too, and their attitudes and behaviour often cause heartache, stress, and worse. There is increasing evidence that many alternative therapies have real value when combined with mainstream therapies, but there is very little evidence that these alternative approaches are effective on their own.

Most important, there is evidence that patients who are better informed and active participants in their treatment have better outcomes, as in increased survival rates and/or enhanced quality of life. Clearly, the healthcare system and the people who work in it need patients like this. Fortunately, a few cancer centres and foundations have engaged "cancer coaches" to help patients to navigate the admittedly bewildering and sometimes scary healthcare maze, to become better informed and more responsible partners in their treatment. More about that later in this piece.

I Found out Who My Friends Were – Support Systems

My support system was extensive and very surprising. I do not see myself as a gregarious person or someone with an extensive network of friends. Yet people kept appearing, offering to help in the most varied and useful ways: they drove me to treatments, they prepared food, they called, they visited, they wrote, they provided nursing care, they helped me navigate the healthcare system, and they did many other useful things.

We thought we knew who our friends were and who would help. What we found was that some people on whom we thought we could count simply disappeared; on the other hand, many people who we didn't know well helped a lot and have since become good friends.

I learned a lot from the people who supported us and from those who didn't. Why did some "friends" disappear rather than help? How many of them were merely afraid of me as a mortality mirror reminding them of their own certain death, a death they couldn't face? How many simply didn't care to engage with weakness? Believe me, I was weak. How many were simply so self-involved that dealing with me wasn't an option? That certainly seemed to be the case with some business associates, rats who fled my apparently sinking ship. Some actually tried to re-engage me after I became "better."

Those who helped taught me more. Each one gave up a part of his or her life to help. There was no pay, no one's career was enhanced, many were inconvenienced. Yet each person helped consistently, excellently, reliably, with a sense of humour and dedication. So, what was in it for them? Are helping others, good relationships, love, discipline, kindness, forgiveness, battling bad things with courage and a sense of humour rewards in themselves? Undoubtedly, there was something else for each person, too. Some learned about food, some were able to use skills like nursing, some found our conversations and written exchanges worthwhile, some found Annie and me courageous and liked being part of that. All reported that helping was a positive experience, one they would happily repeat. If these simple things are so satisfying, why is there so much bad stuff going on in the world? Do we need to know people before we can feel good about helping?

Did I mention the importance of a sense of humour? I could not have done without it. In my experience, it had to be combined with a dead sober acceptance of the situation, a diligent eye on my care, and a relentless pursuit of knowledge about the science and treatment practices and protocols surrounding my disease.

Support comes in a variety of flavours. In my case, all of them were delicious.

Drivers

Annie and I had initially assumed that she would drive me to my radiation treatment every day. This entailed at least an hour of her time four days a week, and two or more hours on the fifth day, when I had my consults with the doctor and dietician. This represented a big dent in her day, as Annie was already trying to run our business, deal with my bizarre food requirements, and have some semblance of a life of her own. Almost magically, people offered to chauffeur me to my treatments. I wound up with four regular drivers, one for each day of the week, except Friday. Apart from one or two occasions, each person drove every week for seven weeks. On those days, I had back-up drivers pre-arranged. Annie continued to drive me to the Friday appointment since that was when we saw the doctor.

The drivers and I shared a very intimate experience. Over the course of the treatments, I became more tired, more "sun burnt," less able to eat or speak. I probably became noticeably weaker and they all remarked on my "Christmas ham" look after each treatment. While I was in the treatment room, each driver sat in the waiting room, which was filled with people from all walks of life with different forms of cancer, at different stages of development. In some cases, the effects of the disease were horrific. My friends saw these people, how they handled their physical trials and fears, their families and friends, how the clinic worked, how I changed over the course of treatment.

I knew two drivers well at the beginning of treatment. The other two, one a well known politician, the other a scientist / engineer / entrepreneur, surprised me by offering to take me to treatment. At the end of the treatment, I thanked each driver; to a person each of the drivers thanked me! We developed very strong bonds that survive to today, some two and a half years later.

Food

As the treatments progressed, I became increasingly unable to eat solids, to taste anything, to tolerate spices of any kind, to swallow. The inside of my mouth was burnt to a crisp, blood was continuously trickling down my throat, I had no saliva, I developed fungal infections, and I had to drink strange concoctions to keep my mouth moist and free of gunk.

The environment in my mouth was constantly changing. Something I ate happily one day I could not tolerate the next. Add to this that I had to eat at least five times per day, just to keep my weight up and that I tried to eat in a way that did not endanger my cardio health. In short, I was a joy to cook for.

I've already mentioned that I ate by texture, not taste. I came to have favorite textures, some surprising and unpredictable. For example, I liked many purees, lumpy soups (small lumps) and mashed stuff. You already know that I hated ice cream. I only tried it once. Yuck!

Indefatigably, Annie researched and prepared healthy alternatives for me to eat or drink . . . for about four weeks I could only drink. This was an enormous task, and people pitched in to help. Soups, drinks, whole meals made to Annie's specs appeared; our freezer filled up, and I emptied it all into the bottomless pit of my stomach. Everything that people prepared was healthy. Although I was too weak to participate, I saw the amount of effort that went into preparing these concoctions. Yet people took time out of their busy lives to prepare them. Quickly, we had a food support system that was organized and complete. Some people made soups, some made fancy mushes, some shopped, others used food from their gardens. Needless to say, we have some new friends as a result of this and some people with whom our relationships have become less intimate.

Visiting, Calling, Writing

Friends who live in other cities wrote regularly. Not too much, but enough for me to know that they care and that they found my emails valuable. I was able to renew and sustain a variety of relationships. We wrote to each other about many things: how to deal with cancer (some people also had it or were caring for people with cancer); good jokes; family and practical everyday things; the quality of healthcare delivery and policy and how to improve it – an acquired taste for some but now a passion for me; facing mortality; the spirit; what matters in life; and other "big" topics.

People called. I've lived and worked in a lot of places, so the callers were from all parts of North America. Some called weekly for many weeks. Some called less often, but their calls were no less appreciated. These calls were important because they immersed me in worlds and perspectives that were bigger and different from the routine of my day-to-day shuffle around the house and to treatment programs. In the calls, we chatted about stuff that was going on in the lives of my callers, discussed weighty topics, laughed, generally hung out, and, of course, talked about my condition. I liked that no one was maudlin, some were searingly funny, and all were able to deal with my cancer matter-of-factly without dwelling on it. A few people who called also visited.

I had regular visitors, too. Not too many since Annie acted as a gatekeeper. She was concerned that my energy would be sapped by too many visits and perhaps by visits of the wrong kind. One couple once brought a small bouquet of a variety of flowers that I especially like. Since they were not from a florist, I remarked that they must be from my visitors' garden. "Oh, no," she said. "They were growing in a lot. He [the husband] climbed a fence to get them. He has a hole in his pants to prove it." "He" is in his seventies and quite respectable. The picture in my mind of him scaling a fence and ripping his pants to get me some flowers is an image I won't easily forget.

I had two special visitors, friends who are former cancer nurses. Both were specialists in neck and thoracic cancers. One is now a real estate agent and the other is a yoga teacher. Both came to assist with aspects of the recovery for which Annie wanted help.

The Most Important Support

Annie was my most important support. Emotionally she was a rock; for the members of the support system, she was an organized, kind, and firm manager of their gifts; for my family and close friends, she was glue and a calm source of balanced information; for me, she was everything positive, everything I needed.

Some things I will never forget: The look on Annie's face, the sound of her voice and the touch of her hand when she first saw me after the operation. The same as when we fell in love, the same as when we say goodnight or good morning. Kind, loving, necessary: the same every day we have together.

My son's tenderness and the way he bravely masked his shock at my appearance when he came to visit on Father's Day, less than two days after the neck operation.

My family doctor's steadfastness throughout this whole journey: from her initial suspicion of an infection to knocking down doors to get me seen during the diagnostic process to her ongoing support.

My grandson who gently touched the scar on my neck soon after the surgery and said: "I'm glad they took that chicken bone out of your neck," He was three and half years old, had been told nothing about my disease, but apparently had noticed the lump on my neck caused by one of the tumors.

In many ways, my supporters were my best coaches. Every word, laugh, encouragement, normal interaction, or heroic intervention were teaching moments for me, helping me to remember to put one foot in front of the other and to get as much out of every moment as I could.

Helping Others Surf the System

In my journey through the health care system, I have dealt with senior and junior practitioners in their fields. Many of these people are admirably dedicated, caring, and knowledgeable. I have, however, run into others who aren't, who care more for technique or following rules than for patient well-being. Some even parade around with insufferable arrogance. All live within the bubble world of the healthcare system, with its rules, procedures, and sometimes stupid bureaucracy. Dedicated or not, caring or not, they need partners, non-medical partners: to help where the system hamstrings them, to offer new perspectives, to gently puncture the bubble when it behaves like a boil that needs to be lanced.

Examples abound. Consider this: doctors live with an almost feral fear of liability. It influences their decisions and the guidelines and procedures they follow. The problem is that slavishly following guidelines is not always the best medicine, nor does it encourage cautious creativity when the need for it is indicated. My case is an example. I would have been diagnosed quickly and my cancer would have been caught at an earlier stage had I had an excisional biopsy first or immediately after the inconclusive fine needle aspiration. To a person, the doctors knew from clinical experience and from the results of x-rays, ultra-sounds, and the like that I probably had cancer. Yet they wasted time and money with testing that took another few months to complete, and resulted in the cancer progressing. I could fill pages with other examples.

I volunteer on a committee that works with key cancer providers in the healthcare system. These are the decision makers in the cancer establishment in my community. Many of them are also senior practitioners in their fields. The committee, which is a partnership of medical professionals and laymen like me from the community, sets policy, program, and quality guidelines for a foundation that provides a range of support for cancer survivors, their caregivers, and the cancer community in general. The idea is that professionals from within the system and from the community cooperate in designing and setting standards for these programs. This foundation finances clinical research, something that is not funded by the system in my community; it makes diagnostic and treatment available in regions surrounding Ottawa so that patients can be served close to home; it buys and donates diagnostic and treatment equipment. One of its most important activities is a centre that offers programs that supplement what is available in the healthcare system. These include yoga, and T'ai Chi, and other exercise geared to the abilities of the participants; nutritional advice and cooking classes; stress management; naturopathy; music and art therapy; humor and laughter groups; bereavement support; and a number of other programs, including coaching for patients and their caregiver family members.

I practice a form of informal, non-prescriptive coaching. My clients come by word of mouth; I don't advertise. I suppose it is a natural outgrowth of my background: at one point in my life, I practiced as psychotherapist and counselor using non-prescriptive methods.

My coaching experience began quite unexpectedly between the end of my radiation treatment and the radical neck dissection. A friend called and asked if I would speak with a guy who was facing a cancer diagnosis. He was quite freaked out, but also a proud officer in the military. He was ashamed to tell people at work. So I called and chatted with him and his wife. I won't go into the specifics, but we spoke a few times about various aspects of the cancer journey and the healthcare system. I thought nothing more of it, although I did call to see how he was doing.

Then, another person called and asked me to do the very same thing for one of his friends. Then another person called with a similar request. I soon realized that there is a large need for helping people deal with their personal issues, become informed about their disease, and intelligently navigate the healthcare system during the diagnostic, treatment, and either recovery or end-of-life phases of cancer. I now do this when I am asked.

This isn't counseling. Many cancer centres offer counseling. Coaching definitely needs to be somewhat independent from the healthcare system. Some of the work is to help patients whose interests somehow clash with the system (e.g., shortcutting protocols, etc.). People working in the system or who are beholden to it may not be willing to do that. Sometimes I am a teacher; sometimes I simply help people navigate the system and become partners in their treatment.

I don't tell people what to do but rather encourage them to find their own way and make their own decisions. I support self-discovery and self-help by providing a safe and supportive environment, treating every case as unique, listening very carefully, and respecting each person's temperament and situation. I try to pose informed questions and provide sources of information. It doesn't hurt that I'm a cancer survivor, have been through radiation and major surgery, and treat the cancer journey in a compassionate yet matter-of-fact manner.

Now, a new breed of professional, called a "cancer coach," has appeared. Guidelines for coaching are being drawn up, distinctions between coaching and counseling are being made, and competing bodies are now certifying cancer coaches. I suppose that this professionalization of cancer coaching is inevitable, especially given the current societal mania for certification. There is an undeniable need to help people and their families deal with cancer, and I'm sure that some of these coaches will do so. When the dust settles, the jostling for recognition calms down, and the politicking reaches a reasonable level, professional cancer coaching will be an honourable and important profession. The Ottawa Regional Cancer Foundation is a Canadian leader in developing and deploying cancer coaches.

Yet I want to hold out for informal coaches, too – people who are good supports, good mirrors, understanding helpers. I urge you to support cancer patients and to help their families. You may not be able or want to do what I do, but support comes in many forms. We all have gifts. What are yours? Offer them to people with cancer and their families. You can drive, you can cook, you can call, you can write, you can visit people, you can do yoga, perhaps you can play music, perhaps you can draw, and so on. Whatever you do, it can be a form of coaching if you do it with kindness, sensitivity, humour, and realism. The best part is that you'll likely get more than you give.

Final Thoughts

My story is not remarkable, courageous, or special in any important way. It is simply an account of one person who has lived with cancer and who has a good chance of long-term survival. Thousands of people deal with cancer every day. Even more people – family, friends, caregivers, healthcare practitioners – support them in some way. Patients suffer, undergo treatments, find strength they didn't know they had, face fears, mend or deepen relationships, find the importance of love and hope in life.

A good number die.

A few come out relatively unscathed, but most survivors live with disabilities caused by treatments like chemo, surgery, and radiation. Although they are effective, many treatments are truly barbaric.

In my case, radiation has virtually eliminated my saliva and so I must continuously sip water and go through various rituals to keep my mouth and teeth disease free (a job usually done by saliva). I have lost about 60% of my taste and I am very sensitive to even moderately spicy foods, which literally burn the inside of my mouth. I cannot eat foods that aren't "slippery," and even then, I have to drink a lot while eating. For "normal" meals, I often have a side of olive oil or plain yogurt to mix with food to help me get it down. I used to like wine, which I drank in moderation. Now the taste of wine is repulsive.

I cannot spend much time in the sun. I received so much radiation to my neck and parts of my head and shoulders that there is a real danger of skin cancer caused by exposure to the sun. I used to spend a lot of time biking and working outside. Now, I do so only in the early morning and late afternoon and I slather on sun protection even on hazy days.

From nerve damage during surgery, I have permanent problems with one shoulder and my shoulder blade; I also cannot feel all of the left side of my face, which is partially frozen. I have a crooked smile, and have to be careful when I articulate words or people misunderstand what I've said. My neck doesn't move as well or as freely as it used to. I can't sing very well anymore, a big loss for me – maybe not so big for people around me.

Yet, my problems are minor compared to what others have gone through, and what they have to live with. The long term effects of chemo can be devastating. Chemo-related disabilities can increase over time and can be quite severe; organs can be permanently damaged. People who have had the same operation as me have had parts of their jaw removed, had nerves severed or removed, and have suffered other effects that resulted in serious disfigurement. People have lost their stomachs; have become incontinent; have suffered deep vein thrombosis; have suffered thrombocytopenia (low platelet count), which can produce aneurysms; bones have been deformed; limbs have been amputated; voices have been lost; eating has become an unpleasant necessity. This is only part of a very long list.

Cancer is a modern epidemic. All indications are that the incidence of cancer will increase before it decreases. It will permanently mark many lives. The chances are very good that yours is one of them. Cancer will stalk all age groups, all lifestyles, and all walks of life. It will kill many of us.

In 2011, Canadians lost a remarkable public figure to cancer. No matter what you thought of Jack Layton and his policies, he left us with a prescription for dealing with cancer that I know from first-hand experience to be good and true:

> *"You must not lose your own hope. Treatments and therapies have never been better in the face of this disease. You have every reason to be optimistic, determined, and focused on the future. My only other advice is to cherish every moment with those you love at every stage of your journey . . . love is better than anger. Hope is better than fear. Optimism is better than despair. So let us be loving, hopeful, and optimistic."*

Laugh, love, be kind, be realistic, and pursue your passions.

Fear and despair are debilitating and isolating: they make us angry, unhappy, depressed, closed up. Who needs that? Hope, love, and compassion open us, make us happy, help us to laugh, to learn, to appreciate the moment, and, importantly, to get through the tough stuff. It's not always easy to face down fears. People with cancer need the kind of support that helps them help themselves.

Oh, the Places We'll Go

Lisa Newman

Part One

We Go to Cancerland

After thirty plus years as a hospital social worker, I thought myself pretty familiar with health care and with professional caregiving. And on a personal level as well, I thought I knew a lot about being a caregiver. After all, I had parented three children born within five years and successfully weathered teething, toilet training, schooling, even adolescence, and now I could enjoy three responsible adult offspring. All my experiences of caregiving as a social worker or a parent, however, paled beside the responsibilities I was to assume as a caregiver to my adult loved ones. As the saying goes (in so many languages the world over), "small children, small problems."

My induction to adult caregiving came very late one Christmas eve when my bedridden, elderly mother began to have trouble breathing and was in distress. I realized that she needed more help than I could give her and that it was up to me alone to connect her to the healthcare system.

Calling our GP – who had faithfully looked after all of us for 40 years – was out of the question: like so many crises, this one was happening outside office hours and on a holiday. Mom, a frail 93 year old woman, had for the last while been unable to speak, let

71

alone participate in decision-making. Her late spouse (my father) and her whole family was deceased; my only sibling, my brother, was thousands of miles away in Mexico. I was on my own with this one.

The housecall doctor who came in response to my call was young, earnest, and quite thorough. He examined Mom, shook his head, and declared "we" were sending her to the hospital emergency department.

This was one scary moment. Everything I knew about hospitals from my own hospital career told me that whatever else was going to happen that night, Mom should definitely not go to the emergency department. By going into that potentially dangerous environment, she would be risking infections, falls, and worse. And there was no one but me to make this decision. I was frankly scared at the huge responsibility I felt I had to take on, and I have never felt more alone.

I took my courage in my hands, announced that "we" were not sending her to emergency, and so "we" would have to make a different plan. "So now what can we do?"

The young doctor looked stumped and not a little put out.

"Well," I continued, "if she were to go to hospital, what exactly would you do for her there?"

"Easy: take an X-ray of her chest. She is breathing so shallowly that I cannot hear if her lungs are clear or not."

"And after that?"

"Well, if the X-ray shows she does have an infection in her lungs, I would order an antibiotic immediately."

I tried to imagine it: this treatment would be given after Mom would have been lying cold and miserable on a thin stretcher mattress in the emergency corridor for some hours. She certainly would not rate a high priority as compared to the heart attacks, car accident victims, and so on that are the emergency's regular clientele. In the worst case, she might be regarded as a "GOMER" (Get Out of My Emergency Room) by the staff, something no one wants to be.

I took another deep breath: "How about you just prescribe the antibiotic now?" I knew, in fact, that he would not want to wait the several days to take cultures of whatever was growing in her lungs. "I can then just race up to the local all-night pharmacy and get her the drug. She will have her first dose within the hour and stay safely in her own bed, not exposed to any ER risks."

And that is exactly what "we" did, after he laboriously noted on the chart we kept at home, "daughter refusing to send patient to hospital, against medical advice"; In other words, his ass was covered.

By the time I was able to consult the family doctor almost a week later, Mom was making a nice recovery on the antibiotic; he reassured me that I had done absolutely the correct thing. In his words, "'we' don't want her to go to emergency!"

Flash forward to a Saturday night in Manhattan, May 2003: my husband David and I had just completed a strenuous hike of several days up the bank of the Hudson River with our group of hiking friends, and I was eager to go out on the town. What a treat: we did not get to New York often, and I had visions of theatres, interesting restaurants, or just strolling the avenues. But all David wanted to do was lie around our hotel room and sleep. This normally very energetic and social 66 year old man, usually full of beans, could not be enticed to leave our room. Frustrated, I very reluctantly settled down to read a book.

Back in Toronto, David's malaise continued; he remained listless and low in energy, not at all like the hyperactive husband I knew and loved. Other puzzling signs appeared, like an angry red rash on his shins that the dermatologist David consulted did not know what to make of. While in hindsight, these were hugely important events, we did not pay too much attention to any of them at the time since we were in the middle of moving into our newly restored house, something we had been planning and working toward for over a year.

But a couple of weeks later, settled now into the new house, David was still feeling no better and so he made an appointment with our family doctor, Dr. A. (Dr. A. is an excellent family doctor, a senior member of the family medicine department at a large teaching hospital who has served all our family very, very well over many years). Dr. A. herself was not available that day, and the colleague filling in for her listened to David's symptoms and ordered a number of tests, including one for liver function. The liver function tests are not routine, but when asked later, the doctor said he just had an inkling that this malaise of David's had been "going on too long." When his liver enzymes came back as being out of whack, a CT scan was ordered, and after a week or so, David was duly scanned. Meanwhile at home, we resumed unpacking our many boxes, arranging the furniture, putting books on the shelves, and hanging pictures. Then Dr. A. called and asked us to come in at the end of her clinic on Thursday.

And so it was on June 19 at 1:15 pm that we were sitting in Dr. A.'s office to get the result of the tests. Though she had asked me to come along with David, I still thought we were dealing with something like hepatitis. I still did not think that this could be something life-threatening, until, sitting there in her office and feeling completely numb, I heard myself repeating the words she had just uttered: "David has a 2 cm growth on the head of his pancreas." Those twelve words changed our lives forever. Like the captain of a ship run onto the tip of an iceberg by mistake in the dark, we knew we were facing something huge and awful but could not make out in detail the looming disaster ahead of us. We felt very small and felt an urgency about preparing but were not sure how or what we needed to prepare. We felt numb, as one who is cut and sees their own bleeding without yet believing it or feeling pain.

I was surprised when Dr. A. asked us to please keep her informed of David's progress, explaining that the communication links with "Cancerland" were not always good and that she often lost track of her patients once they entered cancer treatment, even within the same hospital. We left her office with the promise of an appointment to be made for David to see Dr. G., a well known cancer surgeon at the hospital. Feeling shaken and shell shocked, we walked around the block trying to take in the fact that our whole lives had just changed irrevocably. David spoke of some regrets of his life, things that now would never be; I stayed silent, pondering how my own life was about to change drastically.

Waiting for Surgery

Our appointment with the surgeon followed within a week. We were glad to hear that he thought he could resect (surgically cut out) the tumour, but the soonest that surgery could be scheduled was July 21, over a month after David's growth had been found. Did that month's delay allow the tumour to grow beyond being resectable? My cousin, a U.S. surgeon, kept calling and inquiring about the delay in getting David to surgery; I believe there would not have been such a delay had we been living in the U.S. A later CT scan did show that in the two and a half months since David's initial scan, his tumour had increased in size by over 50%, from 2.0 to 3.5 cm.

On the one hand, David was lucky that the tumour on his pancreas was found early and before it caused pain (by which time it is usually too late to do much), but on the other hand, he was unlucky to have presented himself as a patient for surgery in late June. Why was this unlucky? Because all hospital house staff (doctors in training, including interns, residents, and fellows) move to their next rotations on July 1 each year; this administratively efficient system has clinical consequences since the mass migration of doctors cuts many hospital services to a minimum for the last week of June and the first week of July. In addition, the new doctors coming in don't yet know the new hospital routines, their new colleagues, and so on. Having worked as a social worker in teaching hospitals for thirty years, I myself would routinely advise friends and family to avoid going to hospital in July, and now this was exactly what David was about to do. (For suggestions on how to relate to the bewildering number of healthcare professionals, please see **Chapter 3: System Navigator** in Part Two below, p. 115).

We were very busy in the weeks waiting for surgery, researching everything we could find in books or on the web about pancreatic cancer and speaking with relatives, friends, and friends of friends who had cancer experiences to relate and suggestions to offer. David prepared a summary of his finances, which he shared with me and with Steve, his best friend and executor. We visited the cottage for a long weekend before surgery, swam, and went for long walks on some of our favourite country roads. And, daunted in advance by the volume of calls from our many friends and relatives wanting updates, I signed up online to build and manage our own website, where I would be able to enter updates almost daily and where wellwishers could post messages of support to us. The website was a godsend in many ways. It fulfilled the original purpose of relieving me from repeating the same (often painful) information over and over. Even more helpful, it created a virtual community where David could share his musings about everything from the history of the ancient world to the healthcare system to contemporary politics. (For tips on setting up your own website, see **Chapter 5: You Too Can Be a Website Manager** in Part Two below, p. 124).

The many messages of support we received really buoyed David's spirits; as he wrote,

"Listening to and reading your beautiful, supportive, loving, prayerful and funny voicemails and emails gives me the best of both worlds: I get to hear my eulogies but without being committed to the funeral. Actually, now that I have heard the eulogies, I am going to try to duck the funeral."

Loneliness, too often the sick person's companion, makes everything seem worse; a loving caregiver and loyal friends can mitigate that. As David later wrote on our website,

"I couldn't handle both illness and isolation. I am thriving, partially from Dr. B's aggressive chemo and the faithful care of Dr. R. and staff, partially from the experimental drug, more than partially from Lisa's constant attention and optimism and partially from your wide and deep support. I could not do this alone."

(**Chapter 2: Being There** in Part Two below, p. 111, underlines the importance of a caregiver's presence).

Surgery and Aftermath

David was admitted bright and early the morning of surgery; he was in good spirits as they wheeled him into the operating room. We were told to expect an eight-hour operation, so I headed home to busy myself with cooking and housework rather than sitting and waiting. Within a couple of hours, there was a call from the surgeon, who told me that David's tumour was located right on a key vein, and though he tried very hard, it was not possible to remove it all. He explained that if he could not remove it totally, then it was better to leave it in place. The definitive pathology report would take a couple of weeks, he said, but the tumor did appear malignant. The only good news was that the lymph node (which had seemed enlarged on the CT scan) did not appear to be cancerous, and this suggested the disease had not spread.

One of the hardest things I have ever had to do in my life was to answer as, still drowsy from the anaesthetic, David sleepily but pointedly asked me, "How did it go, darling?" and I had to tell him that the surgery was not successful.

What next? Probably other treatments like chemo and radiation, but first David would have to regain his strength. This had been major surgery, and the many layers of his tissues that had been cut would need time to knit up and heal.

David stayed in hospital for ten days. I visited daily, but in hindsight, I wish I had remained at his side the whole time. In David's later hospital stays, I simply brought a small mattress and bunked in. That first night, he was kept awake by the ravings of his delirious roommate who was desperate to catch a train home at once. Later, David was moved to his own room, and eventually, his tubes were disconnected and he was able to sit, then to stand, and even to walk – at first with assistance and later on his own.

The nursing care was very good, even though the hospital at the time was under stress of an epidemic (SARS) which severely limited visitors and imposed extra constraints on staff. There were problems initially getting David the right dose of pain medication, and several times, he almost fainted when he stood up, perhaps because of inadequate medication; later, a specialized pain nurse consultant ("Jill the Pill," as she was called, was really very nice) helped resolve things.

The medical care, largely delivered by house staff (doctors-in-training) was more uneven. For instance, it was only as we were leaving that the resident in charge of David's care happened to say, almost offhandedly, "oh, he did have a laxative, didn't he?" When I said that he had not and in fact had not had a bowel movement since surgery, I was handed a packet with the instruction to "give him some of this." Many hours of (avoidable) discomfort for David ensued, until his bowels began working again.

(For tips on advocating for a loved one with hospital trainees and other staff, please see **Chapter 4: Advocate** in Part Two below, p. 121).

There were many points in David's cancer journey where I felt the need to advocate with professional caregivers to ensure he got the particular care I knew he needed. For example, preparing for David's discharge from hospital post-surgery, I had to argue with a bevy of young medical trainees about my plan to take David to the cottage he loved, where he could look out from our light, airy bedroom and see his beloved trees even while he was bedridden. I had found out that Home Care nurses could be arranged to visit him at the cottage daily as needed to dress his wound and that they would even send someone to the cottage to bathe him; I was confident I could manage the rest of his care. With a small local hospital only ten minutes away by car, we would be just as close to emergency medical care as we could be to a hospital from our home in the city.

The difficulties we encountered in trying to arrange for Home Care to dress David's wound at the cottage illustrated how fragmented and uncoordinated our healthcare "system" is. Rather than a system, it is really a collection of silos, each with its own priorities. Advocates are crucially important: patients and families need advocates to bend the system toward their needs, to make it patient-centered rather than provider-centered. Many families and patients are willing to take on the task of advocacy, once they are informed with the information they need to do so. It is not, I believe, necessary to have professional advocates layered on top of an already complex and poorly coordinated "system." Rather, patients and their caregivers need to be better trained to understand and advocate for themselves, providers need to be better trained to inform and listen to patients, and administrators must begin to consider the patient and family perspective as they plan services. (Again, please see **Chapter 4: Advocate** in Part Two below, p. 121, on advocating for a loved one's health care).

David and I spent a calm, healing month at the cottage; the Home Care nurses did indeed attend daily at first but came less often as he got better. At the end of a month, David was almost himself again. We had to use a borrowed wheelchair even to get him into the cottage when we arrived, and for the first week or so, he could only walk the length of the deck, but David's strength slowly increased, and after a couple of weeks, he could do stairs comfortably. Eventually, he walked on a flat road by our favourite nearby horse farm where thoroughbred horses gamboled in green, green grass and came up to the fence to greet us.

In addition to reading, one thing that sustained David's interest even while he could not be very active physically was composing and dictating messages for our website (**Chapter 5: You Too Can Be a Website Manager** in Part Two below, p. 124, gives tips on starting your own website). As David wrote at the time,

"Your messages relax, cure and heal. Lisa started this website pragmatically; I had not the energy and she had not the time to let everybody know every step in this ongoing story. But soon it moved from being peripheral to being central in our lives. We feel a compulsion to read what you write as soon as you write it; we chortle over, or weep over and never less than draw comfort from each message. At the same time, we feel a compulsion to initiate our messages to you and I spend almost as much time making notes of what I want to say as I do reading about pancreatic cancer and the whole complex divided cancer vortex. Of course you know it would be impossible for us to reply individually since, as has been said on this website, being sick really keeps one busy. Because I foresee many points at which I will want to read this whole two-way opus on one site, I would be very grateful if those of you who occasionally send us private emails would consider posting all but the most private messages on this website."

For me as his caregiver, life was full of challenges over and above my usual wifely responsibilities: doing laundry using the cottage's antiquated machine, preparing meals that would stimulate his flagging appetite, finding time to manage our website and dictate daily updates, and so on. It turns out that caregiving is a busy job! (A full list of potential caregiver roles is found in **Chapter 1: Your New Job: Caregiver for Your Loved One** in Part Two below, p. 109).

After Surgery: Now What?

But recovering from surgery was just the beginning, the prelude to the next stop on our (unexpected and unwished for) tour of Cancerland. That next stop was to meet the oncologist and discuss treatment plans. We had an appointment at the cancer hospital for which David prepared extensively, gathering his research, honing his points and evidence, writing and revising as if for a final exam or a legal case. He wrote the oncologist a three-page letter in advance of our meeting, which I am not sure was ever read. Dr. M., the senior oncologist dealing with gastrointestinal cancer, set the tone of our meeting by arriving two hours after the arranged time; during those two hours, we first cooled our heels in the waiting room and then met with his resident for an hour. Our discussion with Dr. M. was understandably intense because we kept suggesting treatment options we had researched and he kept shooting them down for most of the hour that he did spend with us; the only medication he recommended to us was one that we had already learned from our research was well tolerated but not very effective. He informed us David was not eligible for a clinical trial that they were running. And at the end of the hour, as I was in mid-sentence indicating that we had more questions, he stood up and said he had to leave. He did not suggest that I email him our questions, nor that I discuss them with the resident or anyone else. He actually said "If it were me, I might just go to my cottage; if it is not bothering me, I wouldn't bother it." He was suggesting, in other words, that we forego treatment altogether.

Today, I thank Dr. M. in my heart for being so unfeeling and unhelpful. By this time, we had learned in our research that the most innovative work in pancreatic cancer treatment was being done in the U.S., not in Canada; we later came to learn that Canadian oncologists do not see very much volume of this "orphan disease" and the few cases they do see are usually disastrous. They have understandably little motivation for optimism.

And so we concluded that treatment in the U.S. was worth a look. We did not have any idea how to go about this, neither of us ever having had medical treatment outside of Canada, but there was certainly nothing to be looked for here in Toronto. We had been given the name of Dr. B., an oncologist highly recommended by two different friends of ours who did not know of each other; David's experience as a lawyer made him trust this coincidence since both pieces of evidence pointed in the same direction. Back at the cottage, we sprang into action. We called Dr. B.'s office in Brooklyn, New York and arranged to fax them all David's medical information. At the same time, we had telephone consultations with a cancer consultant who integrated alternative and conventional medical treatments (thus avoiding chemotherapy). When, a couple of days later, we had a lengthy telephone conversation with Dr. B., we decided to entrust David's care to him; he arranged for David to be admitted the following week, when he would begin chemotherapy treatment.

Throughout David's illness, we sought information about resources everywhere we could: some of the best information came not from official sources, but from unofficial ones like the internet and other patients and their families. At one point, we discovered a small humanitarian charity that shunned publicity and operated "under the radar"; their highly trained staff and consultants (including, among many others, nurse-practitioners) devoted themselves to helping patients and families connect with needed resources, both locally and abroad. Throughout all our searches, we alone had to sift through and coordinate the masses of information. There was, we learned, no such thing as a healthcare "system": the handoffs among the various facilities are precarious at best, and it takes a dedicated, tough-minded caregiver to coordinate a loved one's care and in effect bend the "non-system" of health care to the loved one's needs. (For tips on being your loved one's healthcare advocate, see **Chapter 4: Advocate** in Part Two below, p. 121).

New York, Here We Come!

The hardest part about getting David to treatment in New York was deciding to do it. Once we made that difficult decision, including the significant financial commitment to pay for his care there, everyone was extremely helpful. Unlike the big Toronto hospital where David had been diagnosed and treated until now, Dr. B.'s hospital in Brooklyn was not a top-flight teaching hospital and was not populated by the many doctors-in-training we were used to meeting. What it did have, however, was a real spirit of caring, evident at once from the top of the organization (like the administrator who came down to explain personally to us why David's MRI was delayed by an hour) to the lowest on the status totem pole (like the food service ladies who very sincerely wished us good luck and success in David's treatment). I have worked in several Toronto hospitals over my thirty year career, but never have I encountered such a positive, caring atmosphere among the staff. Here, everyone seemed aware that their end goal was to help people get well, and everyone acted accordingly. This was not so much the result of a "mission statement" (certainly we have all had our fill of those) but rather a true culture of caring.

Dr. B. (the oncologist) and Dr. A. (his radiation therapy colleague) worked together to initiate David's treatment almost as soon as we arrived. A portacath was inserted surgically into his chest through which David began receiving chemotherapy infusions, and on the same day, he had his first of several radiation therapy treatments. After two weeks of treatment, David had two weeks off back home in Toronto. And just at that time, we came across a timely report of a study whose key finding was that "patients who traveled to receive cancer treatment survived longer than those who were treated within 15 miles of their home." The study, as reported in *The Journal of the National Cancer Institute*, examined the results of over 550 Chicago patients with identical cancer who received identical treatment. About half of them received their treatment in centres away from Chicago. The survival rate among those who left was way, way higher than for those who stayed. In fact, the authors calculated that the survival rate increased 3.2% for every ten miles of distance patients travelled from Chicago. How then to account for this startling distinction? This for sure will be debated and re-examined for years, but one immediate, plausible explanation originates in the distinctions noted below about Stephen Jay Gould. By definition, those who left are more willful, more aggressive, less passive, less accepting of what they are told by the first doctor they visit. Sounds a lot like David and me.

We began travelling to New York for David to receive treatment every other week. Our routine was to leave on an early morning flight, spend the day at the hospital, sleep over at a nearby hotel, and return home at the end of the second day of treatment. Since David loved to eat, we asked around and located an excellent family-run Italian restaurant in Brooklyn where we would have dinner in between. I have fond memories of the crisp white tablecloths, the warm friendly service, and the excellent pasta. We felt on these outings that we had been let out of (cancer) jail.

After a little more than two months of this routine, David's key indicator, a blood test for his tumour marker CA-19, had declined sharply from over 4,000 to 1300. We were ecstatic: we had the cancer on the run and we were winning this war. At the same time, a physician friend of ours offered to check with his oncology colleagues at a suburban hospital to see if they would administer this clearly successful chemotherapy cocktail closer to home. If we did not have to travel to New York for two days out of every two weeks, maybe we could again have something like a normal life. The plan was for David to be infused with the chemotherapy drug close to home (a 45 minute drive away) while still travelling every two months to Brooklyn so Dr. B could monitor David's progress.

The Politics of Cancerland

The politics of cancer treatment seems to include a divide between the teaching hospitals, which must follow the treatment protocols of Cancer Care Ontario, versus the community hospitals whose oncologists have a freer rein. And indeed, the Brampton oncologist consulted by our physician friend agreed to administer Dr. B.'s innovative treatment to David. Why, one might wonder, could this not have happened four months earlier (thereby saving us the efforts and expense of seeking treatment in New York)? Well, it seems that our Brooklyn oncologist was a maverick, and while he was a very innovative and successful clinician, he did not obey the norms of evidence-based medicine to conduct controlled clinical trials and to publish his results. As a result, he was pooh-poohed by Dr. M., the Toronto oncologist, who simply sniffed when we mentioned him back in August. (Other oncologists later confirmed to us that they held Dr. B. in high regard and knew of his successes with pancreatic cancer, but we were to hear of this only later).

The main (and wonderful) thing now, six months after David's diagnosis, five months after his failed surgery, and four months after he had begun chemotherapy, was that not only were we winning hugely against the cancer, but we no longer had to travel every two weeks. Life became a little more normal: we could visit with friends and spend more time just enjoying being at home together. And over the next several months, the crucial tumour marker declined even further to just over 600, about one seventh of its level when David was sickest. Life was looking good.

We continued to spend a lot of time on our website, where David posted his thoughts on many current events and other topics. Though it was originally intended merely as a pragmatic timesaver to avoid me having to repeat myself over and over on the phone, it became somewhat of a lifesaver for David. In his words,

"Writing to you my readers consumes me. I spend most of my time and energy thinking of what to say to you, rather than thinking of my nasty, volatile and aggressive mass. When we are communicating, I think, screw the cancer! So your reading this and getting back to me is no mere gesture; it underpins my resolve and resilience."

The website created a virtual community for us, especially valuable because my intensely social husband did not have the time or energy for much socializing in person while on his cancer journey. And, like any good community, it yielded up helpful information when we asked for it (for example, my request for a good recipe for tuna tartare). (Tips on setting up your own website are found below in **Chapter 5: You Too Can Be a Website Manager** Part Two, p. 124).

Not resting on our laurels, we kept looking for anything else that might help in David's recovery. A naturopath we consulted advised some drastic changes in David's diet, and over time, he was converted from a meat-and-potatoes guy to one much more dependent on vegetables, especially raw ones. (One bit of good news was that raw fish and therefore sushi, a great favourite of David's, were very acceptable on his new diet). We consulted a nutritionist to get even more advice about health-giving foods. And just to be sure, we researched another, additional medication which focused on building up David's immune system. This drug was still in Phase III clinical trials, but after six weeks of filling out numerous application forms and of using every medical connection we could, we received federal approval to purchase and administer this drug to David too. It was administered at the suburban Toronto hospital three times a week and so David still had a lot of travelling to do for treatment, even though it was all "local"; he travelled one hour each way seven out of every ten weekdays, two to receive the chemotherapy cocktail and five more for the additional, experimental medication.

Best Result Yet...But Nothing Goes in a Straight Line

By February, David's tumour marker had declined by a further 60% and was now at 280 (from over 4000 at its height). However, the intense chemotherapy regimen had seriously lowered his hemoglobin (red blood cell count). This anemia made David weak and eventually made him unable to withstand the chemo; another, more long term concern about his persistent anemia was that it could lead to cardiac problems. The oncologists tried to build up his blood using another medication, which succeeded for a while. After a few treatments, that too stopped working, and David had to begin having blood transfusions to bring his blood counts up to normal. However, looking on the bright side (my specialty!) we were glad that the symptoms David was experiencing were all reactions to the treatment, not symptoms of the disease. He had no pain that an aspirin would not dispel, no nausea, and no other symptoms from the cancer itself.

A New Problem

The port that had been surgically inserted in David's chest below the collarbone had been showing problems for a few months as the skin above it began to break down. As the months went on, it became clear that the site was infected and required some heroic efforts and very extensive care of the wound by specialized wound care nurses. Geography continued to present us with challenges: the wound care clinic was about an hour's drive from home and in the opposite direction from the hospital where David was receiving chemotherapy. And so David had to be driven an hour each way to the wound clinic, then an hour each way in the opposite direction to the hospital. On these occasions, he would leave home at 8:30 am and would not return until 4:00 pm. One person opined that David was more likely to die in a car accident than from his cancer.

Still, David was having severe pain in his left chest, presumably from the infected port, that could only be controlled by popping Percosets. Several tests and examinations enabled the doctors to rule out a heart event as a cause. More important, they were also able to rule out metastasis, and so his chest pains were not caused by any spread of the cancer. They also pretty well (though not completely) ruled out a clot or pulmonary embolus. These were the three potentially fatal causes of the pain. David did have pleural effusions (fluid in the left lung) for which he was given two very strong antibiotics. It is a measure of how many different pieces of treatment he was getting, and how busy and distracted we both had been, that we both forgot David needed to take one more drug, an anti-inflammatory called Cerebrex, and he missed taking it for a couple of days. Eventually, the port had to be surgically removed and instead David was fitted with a PICC line, a very thin tube which wound up internally through blood vessels in his arm and shoulder to a major artery near his heart. The PICC line, like the port, was designed to preserve David's veins, which would otherwise become rubbery and inaccessible from repeated puncturing. To keep the PICC line free of clots, it had to be flushed daily with saline and heparin; at first, the home care nurses did this, but later they taught me how to do it. The open wound from which the port had been removed took about a month to heal over, no doubt because of the chemotherapy drugs coursing through David's veins.

As I reflected on all the tasks and coordination required to support David's cancer treatment, it seemed to me a caregiver needs to be quite sturdy and/or have very sturdy supports to manage it all. And speaking of things that needed to be done, I sometimes marveled at how my own energy expanded to meet the challenges of David's illness. One day, I mused that David's illness was in effect the exact opposite of a "jobless recovery" that economists talk about. That is, his recovery generated for me many new jobs: driving to and from treatment, typing entries for our website, sourcing the particular kind of bandages needed for his port, shopping for the particular foods advocated by the naturopath, cooking lima bean soup for him because that is what he feels he can eat, and so on. (And why is it exactly that we do not include such "women's work" in the GDP?) (The many roles of a caregiver are listed below in **Chapter 1: Your New Job: Caregiver for Your Loved One** Part Two, p. 109).

Our Various Metaphors for Cancer Journeys

I often thought of the cancer journey we were on as a metaphorical journey, with some of the benefits and difficulties that I associate with travel. Travel always puts me into a different state of mind. Freed of my mundane daily "to do" list, I am able to perceive my surroundings differently. It is as if I straighten up, look around, and see things I would have missed. I live much more in the moment, and there are many more meaningful moments. I reflect more on my experiences, take time to engage in conversations with strangers – everything seems more meaningful, somehow. In a strange environment, I often feel I can, paradoxically, get to know myself better. I get in touch with a more creative part of myself. I review my own priorities and decide on new directions. Often, I return from a trip with new clothes I like a lot: when travelling, I seem able to shop (not usually an activity I enjoy) very successfully.

So what does any of this have to do with Cancerland? Well, the experience of accompanying David on this "journey" has offered, along with many challenges, some of these same benefits. Since his diagnosis, we seemed to be living in a different context, even when we were in Toronto and not "on the road" in New York. There is much opportunity for talking and thinking of things that in the ordinary pace of life get bypassed. I have heard of people who said they were grateful cancer entered their lives, and I think this is part of what they mean. It is still not something I would wish for, but there are definitely good sides to it. (**Chapter 1: Your New Job: Caregiver for Your Loved One** in Part Two below, p. 109, details the opportunities that accompany the challenges of being your loved one's caregiver).

As for the challenges of this journey, one can compare it to the difficulties of trying to function in a foreign country with strange customs; in Cancerland, we were both in an extended state of hyper alertness, trying to piece together what was happening and to anticipate difficulties. Our days at the hospital, with all their hurry-up-and-wait, were extremely stressful and reminded me of the brain fatigue of trying to speak all day in a foreign language. Our Cancerland journey required us to be alive in the moment, living each moment fully, and at the very same time, to be proactive and strategic as we constantly looked forward and tried to anticipate problems and issues.

For David, however, another metaphor, that of war and conflict, was much more applicable to our experience. As he noted on our website one day about a year into his treatment,

"I feel like a Canadian soldier on Juno Beach on June 6, 1944. Guys are going down all around me, but I just keep going because it is unthinkable not to. I too occasionally dive into a shell-hole to reconnoiter, to gather my courage and my wits, but then I stand up and keep climbing up the beach in the face of the machine gun

fire and the 75mms. By the way, I don't reach for the military analogies; they seem to find me. I open my mouth and there they are."

Flexibility of Treatment Regime

Dr. B. monitored David's illness and treatment very carefully through regular MRI's and blood tests (CA-19). Since we were travelling to and from New York for treatment but living in Toronto, these tests were performed in Toronto in advance of each trip to New York. At times, I had to make a case with the radiology department of our local cancer center, which did not immediately see why David needed an MRI and had offered a CT scan instead. Since Dr. B. had specified he needed an MRI, I bicycled down to the cancer center where I located Maria, the clerk in charge of triaging and managing these referrals. I explained to her our need for an MRI and she very kindly agreed to keep an eye out for these requests and route them appropriately. (Again, tips on being your loved one's healthcare advocate are found below in **Chapter 4: Advocate**, Part Two, p. 121).

When at times Dr. B. had become concerned that David was not making enough progress, he turned his treatment schedule upside down, sharply reducing the duration of treatment, sharply intensifying the chemotherapy, and so on. Now, just over a year after diagnosis, the tumour marker had begun rising again, more than doubling in six weeks, but at the same time, David's blood counts (white and red) were so low that he could not tolerate higher doses of chemotherapy drugs. We returned to Dr. B., who introduced some new drugs into David's regimen; he explained to us his belief that the interactions among the various drugs would amplify their effect since they would potentiate one another. And in fact, the tumour marker (CA-19) over the next few weeks plunged again to about a third of what it had been. But no chance to relax our efforts:

in another six weeks or so, it had doubled itself again; Dr. B. therefore added yet another drug to the chemotherapy mix, one which greatly increased David's fatigue. Our cancer journey was starting to feel like a cat-and-mouse game, with Dr. B. zigging as the cancer zagged, trying to keep one step ahead of it. And just to add more challenge (that we did not need), the new chemotherapy cocktail began giving David serious and troublesome diarrhea, something that is no fun at the best of times but is a serious risk to a cancer patient who is having trouble taking in enough food and keeping his weight up.

The many toxic chemotherapy drugs in David's body seemed to be having a cumulative effect. It was taking him longer to recover from his chemotherapy infusions, and sometimes he felt so low that he postponed the chemotherapy by a week to gather his strength. He even had a serious discussion with Dr. B. in which David proposed that they either space the chemotherapy farther apart or reduce the dosages since he was feeling so fatigued and miserable. But Dr. B. held fast, saying that he would do neither and that the measurement of success was not how David was feeling subjectively but the results he was achieving on post-treatment tests. He said David simply had to hang in until there was a basic improvement in measures like his tumour marker.

With all of this, David and I still considered ourselves lucky to be together and to be fighting this fight together. We made every effort, aided by the many well wishers on our website, to find humour in our everyday lives; here is an example, recorded by me:

"David and I were trying to have a warm embrace this morning...We had to be careful of the sensitive area under his right shoulder where the skin has been breaking down around his implanted 'port,' as well as of his recently broken off tooth which is making his mouth a bit sore, and of course we had to take into account the sizeable bottle of chemotherapy chemical which he has

had to wear, attached by tubing to his 'port' for the last 24 hours. We are thinking of registering for some courses with the Cirque de Soleil acrobatic troupe..."

(An important rule in the cancer wars: catch humour wherever and whenever you can; **Chapter 10: Humour** in Part Two below, p. 146, emphasizes the power of humour as a healing tool).

And so the months wore on. We continued going to New York every two weeks, most often flying but driving when the weather and David's energy level allowed. While driving could be tiring and take a long time, the intermittent delays and problems of air travel were very disconcerting. More than once, we found ourselves marooned in the airport, unable to take off; once or twice, we were stuck on the tarmac with no food and no prospect of getting any. And so the driving option was attractive, at least in good weather. With time, we also found a pleasant hotel to stay in near the hospital, which cut down our time commuting within New York City. They gave us the Bridal Suite there, which caused some giggles.

A year and a half from diagnosis, David's tumour appeared about the same size on MRI as it had been at diagnosis, but some of what that image showed may have been dead tumour cells, not active disease. David's tumour marker, CA-19, again declined to a fairly low value (about 350) but it seemed this was at the cost of his feeling weak, having little appetite, and suffering from diarrhea (which was becoming a chronic problem). Not surprisingly, he was therefore once again losing weight. I expended a good deal of energy enticing David to eat, cooking things I knew he liked, or ordering dessert when we went out (even if I did not really want it) in the hopes he would be tempted to try it.

Sources for Optimism in Cancerland

We were very fortunate to encounter many of the goodhearted, generous people sprinkled through our heavily overburdened healthcare system whose responses to David's needs were caring, effective, and efficient. They encouraged and comforted us and gave us more strength for the battle we were fighting.

We were well aware that pancreatic cancer was considered one of the nastiest cancers, generally devastating its victims and leaving them for dead after a brutally short illness. But we held on to our optimism in every way we could. One organization that was very helpful to us was PanCan (short for Pancreatic Cancer), the only organization specifically dedicated to pancreatic cancer. It was started only a few years ago by two energetic young women in the U.S., both of whose fathers had died of the disease. PanCan has done a remarkable job disseminating information, raising money for research into pancreatic cancer, creating support networks, and advocating for more research dollars for this awful disease. As they say, "the science follows the money," and they have succeeded in greatly increasing the total for National Cancer Institute grants to study pancreatic cancer in the U.S. Pancreatic cancer is considered an "orphan disease" because of the small numbers who are diagnosed with it. And since many die terribly soon after diagnosis, there is no body of patients and families to advocate for more research and treatment, unlike for other more chronic diseases. At the moment, there are only ten full-time researchers in pancreatic cancer in the whole U.S., far, far fewer than the numbers engaged in investigating the "biggie" cancers like breast, colon, lung, or prostate.

While the number of sufferers of pancreatic cancer is much smaller than, for example, breast cancer, the number of deaths is very high, which makes a compelling case for more research. I attended several PanCan conferences, and David and I went together to one in Los Angeles where he was very encouraged to meet people who were twelve and more years from their diagnosis of pancreatic cancer and still alive and well. One point that was emphasized was the importance of getting a second opinion, which reminded me of the wonderful Bloch Cancer Foundation, founded by Richard Bloch (also the founder of H&R Block), who lived 30 years after his cancer treatment and died recently of heart failure in his late 70s. Amazingly, the first oncological opinion he had received had given him 90 days to live. (**Chapter 7: Information Manager I** in Part Two, p. 134 below, gives tips on how to research information about your loved one's condition and potential healthcare resources).

Another source of comfort came from our hardheaded consideration of statistics, for which we thanked the distinguished evolutionary biologist Stephen Jay Gould, whose inspiring thesis, outlined in an article titled "The Median Isn't The Message," debunked the power of statistics to predict the future. Gould lived for nineteen years after being diagnosed with a "fatal" stomach cancer that he initially was told would soon kill him. In that time, he wrote all his great books, including his last one on baseball. He pointed out that science's need to categorize does help lead to major treatment advances for huge numbers of patients. However, these categories cannot tell you the outcome for any particular individual. Who is to say where a single person is located on the curve of the survival data for his or her disease? Gould shredded the whole basis of medical medians and averages as statistical abstractions that assume Mother Nature creates rigid categories of conditions around which revolve a few exceptions. He said the opposite is true: the exceptions are just as normal and are an inherent part of all natural conditions.

What we decide is normal is a purely abstract construction made up by the human mind; in fact, nature itself is multivariant and complex. And so, "the normal is almost never." If the national unemployment rate in Canada is, say, seven percent, in fact it is not seven percent anywhere. It is, say, twenty percent in rural New Brunswick and, say, one percent in Calgary. Similarly, the 95 percent fatality rate for pancreatic cancer includes the obese, the passive, the newly divorced, the depressed, or those desperate to be reunited with lost loved ones on the other side. The 95 percent figure does not segregate out as a separate group those who are willful, sceptical about what the doctors tell them, aggressive, and used to solving challenging problems. We should not mistake a statistical abstraction for a prediction, particularly not in such a life and death matter as cancer survival. Yet in Cancerland, we often ran into patients and families who considered a figure of a number of months' survival as a death sentence, a sure prediction of their demise. (Again, information is power, and **Chapter 7: Information Manager I** in Part Two, p. 134 below, gives tips on gathering and managing information for your loved one's care).

We Go to the Beach

One very good thing during this time was that we managed to take a Florida beach holiday in between two of David's chemotherapy sessions. While we had been travelling a great deal over the past year and a half of David's chemotherapy, those trips had all been either return trips to and from New York for treatment or sometimes to the cottage to relax. But those trips had done little to alleviate the stress we both felt from David's cancer treatment; we both were feeling the need of some new scenery and a real vacation. We left New York the day David finished one of his regular two-day chemotherapy sessions and flew directly to Sarasota, Florida where we had rented a condo near the beach. David rested a lot and walked the beach when he was up to it; we both basked in the warmth and beauty of the place and enjoyed the many attractions of the nearby town (including the circus museum). At the end of ten full, relaxing days, we flew back to New York for David's next chemotherapy cycle of treatment and then home to snowy (January) Toronto. (Tips for arranging travel with your ill loved one are found below in **Chapter 9: Going to the Beach**, Part Two, p. 142).

David was showing signs of "battle fatigue" as he entered the twentieth month of his epic cancer fight. His clinical markers were still good and his hair was actually growing back in (we were told this was not significant clinically, but it certainly was pleasing aesthetically and good for his self-confidence). But his digestive system, pummeled by all the chemotherapy drugs, was showing signs of stress. The troubling diarrhea reappeared, and it took us a while to realize that it was necessary to preempt it with regular Imodium. Though he had always loved his food and eaten copious amounts of it, a year and a half of chemotherapy had reduced David to someone who had very little appetite and who did not enjoy the taste of food unless it was smothered in spicy sauces. I despaired of keeping his weight up, though I knew this was very important for his recovery. Trying to cast this in a humorous vein, I wrote on our website:

"In my view, I take responsibility for many items in our journey through Cancerland together, and it remains for David himself to take responsibility for drinking 8-10 large glasses of water a day, and for taking sufficient nourishment or supplements into his body. When he doesn't do that, I feel as if he is slowly committing suicide, and I don't feel much inclined to sit around and watch that.

And it was then that we realized something very very important that you will no doubt be glad to know too: there is no way that David is going to die from pancreatic cancer. You see, it is quite clear that out of frustration I will kill him first."

This occasioned a long posting from David on the website in which he gratefully acknowledged the many parts of my job description as his caregiver:

"Here is the partial list of what Lisa does [I am not writing this to 'appease' her; it's been on my mind for a long time]:

• *She has learned from our Home Care nurses how to shoot me up; during every two-week chemo cycle she injects me subcutaneously seven times with Neupogen to rebuild my white cell count. She does this on three consecutive days starting 24 hours after my last chemo drip and again for four consecutive days leading up to the next chemo drip.*

• *She flushes my PICC line, through which my chemo is delivered.*

• *When we travel, she ensures the Neupogen remains refrigerated at all times. This is not so straightforward on airplanes and in hotels. She makes sure we have the appropriate supplies [syringes, vials, alcohol swabs].*

• *She pushes, cajoles and persuades me to overcome my fatigue and move my website ideas, from notes on paper to postings on the website.*

• *She reads extracts of learned articles, as well as the more popular articles and stays up to date on reports from friends at the cutting edge.*

• *She then organizes all this material, and much else beside, into twelve to fourteen large looseleaf notebooks we have, each with about ten dividers. Hey, we were both 'A' students, so we know how to organize huge amounts of material for essays and theses.*

• *She books our endless travel arrangements on the web.*

• *Certain things she does we cannot write about.*

• *From time to time, I get a sore back and left arm that persists for weeks, most recently in Florida; at Lutheran Medical Center she learned how to massage my back and shoulders in many different ways. She does this several times a day both at home and*

*in public. Last Sunday she was doing this for me in a busy ped-
estrian mall in Sarasota, and just as I said to her, 'Darling, you
could charge for this,' a guy came up and said, 'Lady, could you
do me next?'*

• *During my two days of 5-hour chemotherapy infusions,
when I am hooked up and more or less immobile, she runs interference with Finance and Admitting, arranges appointments
with Dr. B. and pushes his staff to make sure he keeps them.*

• *She brings me food and liquids.*

• *She organizes the laptop computer so we both can stay in
touch; I am able to read my market information and market
'rabbis'.*

• *She types all of our website postings and all my email messages.*

• *She has learned who the key people are to speak to [not ne-
cessarily the big people] in booking procedures like CTs and
MRIs; she has discovered how to thread her way through the
almost impenetrable institutional bureaucracy.*

• *She retrieves from the system CDs with copies of all my CTs
and MRIs.*

• *She pushes the Ensure [ugh!] on me and won't let me dress
in the morning until I have weighed in, so she can chart my
weight. When the weight drops, she pushes more Ensure. And
when my weight rises, she still pushes the same amount of Ensure.*

*Above all, from the beginning, she has rarely faltered; she is un-
failingly optimistic and cheerful – except when she is about to
kill me. Then the household gets tense."*

(My own list of the multitude of caregiver tasks is found below in **Chapter 1: Your New Job: Caregiver for Your Loved One, Part Two,** p. 109).

Another New Problem (Due to Treatment, Not Cancer)

At the twenty-third month of his cancer journey, David experienced some new, troubling side-effects of the toxic chemotherapy drugs. His toes were numb and, after a neurological examination, it seemed clear that David's nerves had been damaged by his chemotherapy drugs. This was perhaps a sign from his body that David was nearing the limit of what he could tolerate, and Dr. B. adjusted his medications accordingly. While David's tumour marker numbers still looked pretty good, he was increasingly uncomfortable as a result of the toxic chemotherapy treatment. And each new complication required more visits to doctors and more tests. The latest was an EMG, a specialized neurological test of David's muscles occasioned by the nerve damage in his toes. Would we get to a point where the treatment would be worse than the disease?

There was no question that things were becoming tougher, and it was becoming increasingly difficult to hold fast to our sense of humour. We were inspired, though, by the example of Norman Cousins, who described in *Anatomy of an Illness* how he used humour to heal himself from a dire collagen disease, ankylosing spondylitis. A leading U.S. writer and editor of the 1970s, he reasoned that if Dr. Hans Selye had been right about the negative effects on the body of stress and the unused adrenaline flow from a person's fear and negative emotions, positive effects in the body should be created from laughter. So he had himself moved from the hospital to a hotel suite and, with the help of his Hollywood and his television friends, spent all his days and evenings watching Marx Brothers movies, Candid Camera videos, and the like. He described in his book how laughter helped him achieve sleep, which promoted healing. "I made the joyous discovery that ten minutes of genuine belly laughter had an anesthetic effect and would give me at least two hours of pain-free sleep," he reported. "When the pain-killing effect of the laughter wore off, we would switch on the motion picture projector again and not infrequently, it would lead to another pain-free interval." He made a complete recovery and believes he laughed himself to well-ness. (The importance of humour's health-giving properties can't be overemphasized; please see **Chapter 10: Humour** in Part Two below, p. 146).

David and I would very consciously try to find the humour in events around us. On one occasion, I noted on the website:

"Cancerland doesn't abound in side-splitting humour and hilarity, but sometimes you just have to laugh – if you can.

Mid-day yesterday we suddenly remembered David's long-booked MRI appointment for 9:00 pm at Princess Margaret Hospital downtown. Having come from yet another doctor's appointment, David napped and ate a little and we drove down. Unfortunately, the note that gave us the appointment time did not make clear that in the evening we would have to enter from the rear of the hospital, so we had a long walk around the perimeter of the building, not easy for David with his fatigue. We managed to get there only a few minutes late, and David was ushered in to the MRI suite, in his little johnny-gown, while I waited and dozed. It took a very long time, and I was worried that they were searching for something worrisome, but when the technician brought David back out he explained that, because of David's hiccupping [which the gastric reflux – due to chemo – causes from time to time], they could not complete the pictures and only got half-way through the protocol.

So we got home, tired out by all this, and fell into bed to sleep. One has to stay in good shape, to be sick – it is really challenging!"

101

And, on another occasion, as we were returning from the suburban hospital at a snail's pace through the severe snow storm on our sixteen-lane super highway, David had an urgent need to void and no easy way to accomplish this. In his own words,

> *"I was caught by the juxtaposition of three factors completely out of my control:*
>
> *1. the thousands of millilitres of chemicals and saline I had just received by I.V. [the saline pushes the toxic chemotherapy drugs through my kidneys as quickly as possible, to minimize damage to the body]*
>
> *2. even a sixteen-lane superhighway is a major choke-point in a severe snowstorm in rush hour*
>
> *3. a 66-year old bladder, even though emptied before the trip, has limited capacity.*
>
> *It was excruciatingly obvious to me that my bladder capacity was running out before the road capacity. With only seconds to spare, I remembered one of Churchill's great lines from the War - "making do is the art of doing what you have to do with what you have, not with what you wish you had" [note: none of these words of his have more than two syllables, most have only one]."*

And so David asked me, who was driving, to drink the water in our water bottle, which he then quickly replenished from his own oversupply.

The list of challenges presented by both David's illness and (even more so) his treatment multiplied over time. Diarrhea particularly plagued David in a number of ways: he shed pounds that he could ill afford to lose; he felt unwell and unable to eat; and, perhaps worst of all, he often became seriously dehydrated. At first, we did not recognize this for what it was; we simply noticed that

102

David was lethargic, limp, and unenergetic. Fortunately, the doctor who examined him picked up the signs and ordered that he be given I.V. hydration. David felt better almost immediately. Later, the Home Care nurses provided us with a pole and supplies so that we could hydrate David with an I.V. at home without going to hospital should his hydration became a problem again.

We searched around for medicines that could control the diarrhea. A local gasteroenterologist finally suggested tincture of opium, a time-honoured preparation that did the trick. Though I had some worries about David's potential addiction and images of premodern China flashed before my eyes, these were dismissed in favour of the greater good. But then came the problem of where to buy the stuff. After all, it was a controlled drug, a little old-fashioned and rarely used today, and understandably many pharmacies didn't bother to stock it. Fortunately, a friend knew of a pharmacy where we could reliably get the prescription filled. Once more, information gleaned from friends had been invaluable in navigating the healthcare non-system. (**Chapter 3: System Navigator** in Part Two below, p. 115, has suggestions and navigation tips). We have benefitted from an effective though informal underground network of proactive, caring patients and families and caregivers who share information. And these days, we all have learned that information is power. In this sense, people really can help one another!

Making Memories to Treasure

We insisted on having large family dinners to celebrate all of the Jewish holidays and we manufactured occasions to add meaning to our lives whenever we could. As Viktor Frankl and others have written, it is our uniquely human gift to attach our own meaning to events like serious illness which can seem cruelly absurd. (See **Chapter 11: Making Meaning: Memories You Will Cherish** in Part Two, p. 148 below, for a discussion of the rationale for planning and executing memorable events even during the crisis of life-threatening illness). In May of David's second year of illness, we had a bangup celebration of my 60th birthday, including an excursion with the whole family (nine of us, counting our one year old grandson, Joseph) to a lovely hotel resort and then a great big party at home for our friends and family.

A few weeks later, we held another celebration to mark the two year anniversary of David's diagnosis. We called it "Life Day" and we marked the occasion in a big way. David prepared a lecture on one of the topics he has researched and thought a lot about, titled "Geopolitics, Wars, Geography and History of the Ancient Middle East, and Possible Lessons For Today," which he delivered at our home. I rented chairs, a mike, and a platform, and the whole thing (including a gag heckling interruption by an actor friend) was taped and recorded. About seventy friends and family attended, and we feasted on party sandwiches and drinks afterward.

And not long after that, we were back at the cottage: the third summer of our cancer war. On a couple of occasions during those wonderful, lazy summer months, we extended our stays, deviating from our usual two-week interval to have an extra "feel-good" week at the cottage. David was feeling so debilitated from two years of chemotherapy and the cumulative, miserable side-effects of the drugs. He was also extremely fatigued after each chemo treatment, and above all, sick and tired of being sick and tired. And so these wonderful, sunny extra weeks – with David feeling more and more energetic, walking more than a mile a day, and both of us enjoying a very welcome respite from the chemotherapy grind – were like being let out of jail.

But David (and I) paid dearly for one such break. At the end of August, when his blood was next measured for CA-19, the tumour marker had soared from 610 to 1010. Both the direction and the magnitude of this change were very worrisome. It seemed that the weeks off had in effect diluted David's chemotherapy dose since on several occasions he had been given a two-week dose but did not return till the end of three weeks. In effect, he had been under-medicated. And, in Dr. B.'s words, the tumour is a workaholic, always seeking – and in this instance succeeding – to cause more trouble.

It took almost two months for the chemotherapy to wrestle the tumour marker back down (from 1600 to 764), though it was still about twice as high as it had been in the summer. David's white and red blood counts were extremely low, and the home care nurse injected him with medications for both. As well, he received a blood transfusion at the local hospital. Even with the diarrhea under control, David lost weight all too easily and had a lot of trouble gaining it back.

Cancer and chemotherapy had become such major parts of my own life that I was startled when a very good friend, whom I knew to be a sensitive person, asked me if I ever forgot that David had cancer. No, not for a minute, I answered. This was my not-so-new normal, coming up to two and a half years of challenges, searches, struggles, all in the service of a desperate wish to live.

But cancer was a merciless foe. Having gained some ground over the summer when we let down our guard, it pressed its advantage home. Mid-November was a trip to Los Angeles for the PanCan conference, then straight on to New York for chemotherapy, and then home, with David quite exhausted. But whereas in earlier times, he had bounced back like the energizer bunny, this time, "the comeback kid" was worn out. David got pneumonia, and the tumour increased considerably in size, with its marker rising to over 5,000.

We were never able to make a return trip to New York. Within a couple of weeks, David was admitted to hospital for a last-ditch attempt to nourish him since he was not keeping food down. On the way to the hospital in the ambulance, David – still a big kid – said, "I know it would probably be unreasonable, but on this my first ever trip in an ambulance, I do wish we could have the siren on." The (male) medic said he understood completely, adding "Why do you think I do this job?" But he did not agree to sound the siren.

Upon arrival to the hospital, the gastroenterologist looked through his scope into David's esophagus to see if there was something blocking his food intake, but he found nothing he could remedy. Several other attempts were made to improve David's nutrition, most of them not effective. Initially, he was given an I.V. treatment called Total Parenteral Nutrition (TPN). Later, an N-G (naso-gastric) tube needed to be inserted through David's nose to get nutrition into his stomach. He found the insertion procedure impossibly uncomfortable. And so I leaned over the bed, held his hands and locked eyes with him, and was able to talk him through it while the technician successfully inserted the tube. Once the tube was in place, he began to take in nourishment for the first time in several days. Walking around the gastro ward with the tube taped to his nose, he didn't even look very unusual since a lot of patients there were sporting them, walking up and down the corridor, like at some funny costume party.

At this point, David needed to stay in hospital so he could be stabilized on TPN. We were told the "re-feeding" process in someone like David (whose difficulty swallowing and digesting food over many months had resulted in his under-nourishment) needed to proceed very slowly; experience had shown that rushing to resume feeding someone seriously undernourished can have dire consequences. An example many are familiar with is the concentration camp survivors who gorged themselves on food when they were freed at the end of World War II; sadly, many died, as their starved bodies could not assimilate the nutrition.

Whereas earlier we had defiantly insisted on living as full a life as a cancer patient can – attending art exhibits, operas, and concerts, and socializing with friends and family – now our world had severely contracted to the size of David's hospital room. I stayed beside David around the clock for that month, sleeping on a mattress on the floor. I was able to participate in his care, which was comforting for us both. It was in fact a tender time for us both, and though, in earlier times, David could certainly be demanding and articulate when unhappy, now he was extremely stoic about the dire situation we were in. And so I had a significant role to play as David's advocate, making sure that the hospital's array of staff followed up on and coordinated his various treatments. (**Chapter 4: Advocate** in Part Two, p. 121 below, discusses the caregiver's role in advocating for a loved one's health care).

Friends and family called and visited until David wasn't up to it, and then I had to run interference, blocking visits and phone calls so he could rest. Unfortunately, the hospital phone had no voicemail capability and so we had to just take it off the hook. (Note to hospital planners: install voicemail in patient rooms; it would be a very good way for patients to receive health-giving, supportive messages).

The inevitable happened at the end of December: David became less and less alert, his body swelled up with fluid, he could not speak, and even just breathing became very difficult for him. Over the space of a day, he slipped out of this life; we sang his favourite songs to him as he made the transition since it is believed that hearing is the last sense to go when a person dies.

May his memory be for a blessing.

Part Two

Tips: How to Be
the Best Caregiver You Can Be

I learned so much about caregiving through our Cancerland journey, and the experience made me want to share my knowledge with others. I learned so much from other patients and their families as well as from our own cancer journey, and while I know that everyone's journey (and everyone's personality) is unique to them, I hope that some of what I learned can be useful to others treading a similar path and can make their journeys less arduous. I have divided the following into the various roles that you may be called upon to play as a caregiver to your seriously ill loved one: you may wish to add your own particular roles to the list below.

Chapter 1: Your New Job: Caregiver for Your Loved One

So here you are. A caregiver. This big, new job you just got – the one you never applied for, the one you never really wanted – is challenging, intense, and probably overwhelming. But you can do a great deal to help your loved one get the best care possible. And you are probably very anxious to commit to this job: it is crucially important to you and to your loved one. You really want to get this right!

Some good news: you can write your own job description. You don't have to wait until case managers, doctors, or nurses assign you what you can do; there are many roles you can include in your caregiver job description according to your availability and talents. There are other roles in which your helpers, whether paid or volunteer, can assist you (see **Chapter 6: Coordinator of Volunteers** below). There is much to do. Your loved one will have many diverse needs on the healthcare journey, and these are only some of your possible roles (on top of those you may have already assumed as a family member or loved one):

Activist

Advocate

Bathing Aide

Chef

Coordinator of Recreation and Entertainment

Event Planner, Memory Maker

Healthcare System Navigator

Historian

Information Manager

Letter Writer

Masseur/Masseuse

Motivator

Nursing Assistant

Quality Control Monitor

Relationship Manager

Scheduler

Social Convenor

Tour Operator, Travel Planner

Treatment Team Coordinator

Volunteer Coordinator

Waiter/Waitress

Website Manager

More good news: along with the challenges, there are some hugely positive moments on the difficult road ahead of you. A physician friend who has also experienced the devastating loss of a mate told me early in David's cancer journey, "the only way out is through," and I cannot agree more. By committing yourself to being a caregiver, you are ensuring that, along with an extra helping of life's difficulties, you will enjoy the gratifying experiences of deep friendship and love that you get by giving unselfishly and that will ultimately enlarge you as a person.

You can do this!

Chapter 2: Being There

I became intimately connected not only to David but to David's tumour: I spent so many hours focusing on David's illness and treatment that I was only half joking when I referred to it as "our" tumour. I sometimes found myself in the position of helping David accept necessary care, almost as one would with a child. It helped that I understood the hospital environment, having worked in hospitals for many years.

A troubling instance happened in the last stages of his illness as David was lying, barely responsive, in his hospital bed. We had sadly concluded that there was no more treatment to be given: the disease had won. The feeding tube had been removed since it was not working for him, and the I.V. was unplugged. We were gathered around his bed, struggling to take in this information and accept our imminent loss of David when a respiratory technician bustled hurriedly into the room, inserted her suction pump into his mouth, and vigorously suctioned his airway. David was in no state to protest or even to speak, and so tentatively (assuming she knew something that I didn't) I asked why she was doing this since we had already made the decision to let him go. She was terribly shocked and quickly realized she had come to the wrong patient; she apologized profusely and left the room. Even at this point, with him so near death, I had had a job to do as his caregiver.

What You Can Do

- One of the most useful things you can do for your loved one is just to be there, to show up; your presence is the best present of all.

- As a caregiver, you can lend your memory and your management abilities to your loved one as they are impaired by the illness. You know that as patients, even at the best of times, we often forget to tell the doctor all the items on our "list"; your seriously-ill loved one is even less able to do so. You will do your loved one a great service as you supplement their words by remembering, speaking, or recording for them.

Why Is This Important?

- Being sick is a lonely business; it helps to have company.

- Your loved one will benefit by your being present to discuss their questions and important communications with health-care professionals.

- Political or business leaders always have aides at their sides in important meetings; this support is needed all the more by a sick person who, by definition, has less energy to ask questions or to fully understand the answers.

- You (and your loved one) have a limited amount of time and energy: conserve it! Make sure you are using your energy for the most essential tasks, and delegate whatever you can, so that you can be fully present with your loved one. Even if all you are doing is sitting silently with your loved one, your presence is the greatest gift.

How to Do It

- "Being there" may not sound like much, but if you can be fully present, you will be a great strength to your loved one; the quantity of time you spend as a caregiver may be less important than the quality of giving your loved one full, uncomplicated, attention. This may be difficult to do: you will have many powerful feelings about the process you are going through and about your loved one's diagnosis, illness, and treatment. If needed and if possible, seek out support for yourself, whether from a friend, a relative, a support group, or an online resource. If you are better able to manage your own feelings, then you can better ease the burdens on your loved one, who needs you to be okay not only because they love you, but also so that you can be fully present as a caregiver.

- Do whatever necessary to keep your physical and emotional resources as intact as possible. In this, you are like lifeguards, who are disciplined to keep themselves afloat so they can rescue others and not let themselves be dragged down.

- Keep notes of each visit (see **Chapter 7: Information Manager I.** and **Chapter 8: Information Manager II.** below) so you can refer back to what was said on earlier visits and can coordinate with other caregivers.

- Make sure that all the information about your loved one's history is given to the physician, and make note of any recommendations, rationales for treatment, medications, cautions, and so on.

- Plan ahead for medical appointments by taking notes with you of the questions you want to ask during specific visits and by recording the answers. To this end, you should create a system of keeping track of issues and concerns as they arise. The Agency for Healthcare Research and Quality (part of the U.S. Department of Health and Human Services) has created a helpful guide for formulating questions about your loved one's care, available online at http://www.ahrq.gov/questions.

- In hospital, you can do as much hands on care as you, your loved one, and the staff feel comfortable with. Overworked hospital staff will be glad of your help, especially once they know you understand the limitations or requirements imposed by your loved one's treatment (diet, mobility, medication regimen, and so on). Try to learn the names of the staff and use them to individualize different staff members – just as you and your loved one wish staff to recognize and individualize you.

- You can advocate for your loved one and, knowing the particular details of the illness and treatment, you can catch potential errors. You can point out your loved one's individual needs and any particular family issues to the treatment team.

- Don't be shy about using paid help; it can free you to do what only you can do. If you can afford it, and if hospital policy allows it, consider hiring someone to sit with your loved one while they are in hospital and when you cannot be there. In addition to cleaners, taxis, gardeners, in many large centres you will find a small army of non-profit helpers available for fees geared to income. If you are able to, pay them to shop, cook, or do household tasks; hospital social workers or community information services can help you access these services.

Chapter 3: System Navigator

Entering Cancerland – it was like embarking on an extended trip to a very foreign country. The hospital procedures, the jargon, the many different professionals involved, all created a very steep learning curve for us. Never mind that I had spent countless hours working in hospitals; being on the receiving end, there was so much that we had to learn, and all this under conditions of great mental strain and intensity: David and I were in an extended state of alertness, trying to piece together what was happening and trying to anticipate difficulties – all in a strange environment and in a foreign language. Hospitals are by nature provider-focused, not patient-focused; it is up to patients and their caregivers to orient the system to their needs. On our journey in Cancerland, we had to be both fully alive in the moment, and at the same time, proactive and strategic, constantly looking forward and trying to anticipate problems, issues, and solutions.

As mentioned above, for example, we were faced with a three-week wait for an MRI that David's New York doctor had requested urgently. Our G.P., Dr. B., had followed the accepted procedure by submitting a referral to the cancer hospital; the radiologist there reviewed the referral and decided a (cheaper, quicker) CT scan would do. But our oncologist had specifically requested an MRI, saying a CT scan would not give him the needed information about the state of David's tumour. What to do? I went down to the cancer hospital to talk in person with Maria, the radiology secretary, and to explain our somewhat unusual need. She couldn't have been more helpful, getting the referral processed in a timely way. The combined efforts of hospital staff – Rosa, Andrew, Kristin, and Dawn – turned up an MRI timeslot (a last-minute cancellation), and as we rushed to take it, we felt we had won first prize in a treasure hunt that was combined with an obstacle course.

I kept Maria's number on my contact list and several times had to ask her help to intercept referrals and have them approved for us in a timely way.

Our efforts to make the healthcare system as patient-focused as possible in our case included David's always dressing up to go his clinic appointments; he believed good grooming was critical for a patient trying to elicit the most speedy, helpful responses from the healthcare system. His friend Joan, from personal experience of at least two surgeries, says to her woman friends, "get your hair done, put on your makeup, dress to the nines, and present yourself to the system as someone who is in charge of her life." Look like a somebody and not like so many patients do – broken down, depressed, and disheveled. That way, she says, you can intimidate the nurses and doctors rather than have them intimidate you. And on the subject of grooming and clothes, a friend with a seriously ill husband says she always makes a point of being well-dressed and made up when visiting the hospital because she knew it gave him a lift.

What You Can Do

- The healthcare "system" is not systematic at all. It is really a very loose, complex, uncoordinated array of services, many of them unaware of one another and not at all able to communicate with one another. Hospitals, clinics, and private practitioners may all treat the same patient for the same disease, but each has different funding, different accountability, and most often different information systems. What does this mean for you? Most importantly, reports of your tests or examinations or treatment in one facility may not make it to the hands (or chart) of your other practitioner(s) unless you make sure that happens. It may astonish you to know that while your banking transactions, for example, are shared securely and quickly among many freestanding companies (including those in other countries), your equally – or perhaps more – vital healthcare information may reside on a pen-and-paper chart or an electronic record in a facility that is not accessible to colleagues outside that facility.

- You will find yourself being the "glue" or the thread (to mix a metaphor) that stitches these uncoordinated services together. Think the rigid, centrally directed Soviet economy, unable to match up producers and consumers as efficiently as the free market; producers were left with piles of unconsumed produce and manufactured goods while consumers were experiencing shortages. Informally, the USSR evolved a function for "fixers" who put producers and consumers in touch, facilitated their transactions, and kept the system humming.

Why Is This Important?

- Our healthcare "system" is uncoordinated at best; for your loved one to get the best care, you may need to facilitate your healthcare professionals working together, especially if they are located in different institutions.

- Remember that the system is centred on the needs of providers. It is not patient-focused; it is your task to make it so!

- This disconnect among institutions is even worse if you are crossing jurisdictions to another province or another country.

- You are the expert on your loved one: your information can shape the best decisions for their care.

How to Do It

- *Make Nice*: It is well worth your time to make friends with the clerical staff in your clinic, hospital, or doctor's office. The (often underpaid, overworked) secretary or clerk can and should be your best friend! She (or sometimes, he) has a great deal of power to influence your journey for better or for worse, including shortening or skipping the queue for you, finding you an appointment time where none existed, facilitating your speaking to a doctor, and more. You will score a lot of points with secretaries by simply being courteous and respectful and by making your requests in a polite manner. Hospitals are very hierarchical, originally modeled on armies. Clerks and secretaries are near the bottom of the hierarchy and are too often unused to being treated very respectfully, but they actually do have a lot of power, and things will go better for you if you treat them as such.

- It comes down to the kindness of the good people: they are not easy to find, but when you find them, write down their names and their telephone extensions and write letters of thanks and appreciation to their superiors. Cookies, chocolates, and anything else that will work is not a bad idea. This is not cynical manipulation; it is treating people humanely so that you can expect humane treatment back from them. Even a potentially threatening "Do you mind if I speak to your supervisor?" can be presented in a way which is warm and welcome.

- In hospitals, be sure to check out the roles and responsibilities of various staff members. Not all people wearing white coats are MDs: they might be anyone from a nutritionist to a junior medical student, and their role and rank will determine what they can help you with. Hospital staff are expected to wear I.D. (by all means, ask if you do not see a name tag!), so do not feel shy about asking their profession, their place in the hierarchy, or their experience with a particular illness. In teaching hospitals especially there are many ranks of power and experience, and junior staff rotate often as they learn the different areas of health care.

- You can be a partner in your loved one's health care, and most healthcare professionals will be glad of your involvement as a partner with them.

- Learn as much as you can about the hospital staff schedules, shift changes, etc., so you can be more successful in accessing the staff when you need to. For instance, surgeons are rarely available during the day, as these are their prime operating room hours; you will find them instead early and late in the day, before and after their hours doing surgery. Hospital nurses work either 8-hour or 12-hour shifts, and when shifts change over, nurses are often unavailable because they are occupied doing "report" (passing information about their patients on to the next shift). Social workers, physios, and occupational therapists tend to work Monday to Friday and are rarely available on weekends.

- Like you, healthcare professionals appreciate being treated as individuals; try to learn their names to use next time they are delivering care.

- Find out how the healthcare professionals you need to communicate with prefer to communicate with you and your loved one. Are they more likely to answer emails or phone messages? What hours are you most likely to reach them?

- Always thank people sincerely, and if you are complaining, be specific about what remedy would make it better (e.g., a beeper on loan or a numbering system so you and your loved one do not have to sit for lengthy hours in one spot, terrified of missing your turn.)

- Use the advocacy and support organizations relevant to your loved one's condition: they may have useful ideas and may be able to put you in touch with people who can be very useful to you.

- You may want to seek a second opinion from a physician or team that has particular experience with your loved one's condition; most professionals will not consider this disrespectful at all. A useful website in this regard is http://blochcancer.org/resources/multidisciplinary-second-opinion-centers/.

Chapter 4: Advocate

Throughout our Cancerland journey I often had to advocate for David's welfare, negotiating with hospital billing departments, securing appropriate appointments for MRI scans ordered by his U.S. oncologist, following up on insurance claims, and so on. Sick and growing steadily weaker, David just did not have the strength to fight both the disease and the bureaucracy.

What You Can Do

- As a loving advocate, you can be quite influential in making your loved one's care as good as it can be. No, you don't have to be a nurse or a doctor to do this, just a loving relative or friend. Your unique contribution is that you are *not* a healthcare professional.

Why Is This Important?

- In decision-making about care, the medical professional caregiver's knowledge and reasoning is deductive, from the general body of medical knowledge to the specific signs and symptoms of a particular patient. The more knowledge brought to bear, the better the quality of the decision made.

- Even though you may have never studied a healthcare profession or may never have even been in a hospital, you still have important knowledge to contribute to decisions made about your loved one's care – knowledge that is unique and valuable.

- Non-professional caregivers (*this means you!*) lack professional, medical knowledge but have an important area of expertise that healthcare professionals, by definition, cannot have.

- You know your loved one. You know his or her individual personality, wishes, personal history, state of mind, preferences, supports at home, religious and other values, and so on. The information you hold, while often not captured by the standard outlines for patient assessment, can be crucially important in making decisions for your loved one's care. And only *you* can make sure this information is included in the decision-making process.

How to Do It

- You (and only you) can make the healthcare team aware of your loved one's individual uniqueness, including their wishes for care, their state of mind, and their religious and other values.

- Try acknowledging the individuality of each healthcare worker by acknowledging them by name and by remembering them for the next time they are delivering care; if you treat them respectfully as individuals, they are more likely to treat you (and your loved one) in the same way.

- You can advocate for the care that you know your loved one would want when they are incapable of advocating for themselves.

- On a less dramatic level, you can advocate for measures to increase your loved one's privacy, comfort, and ease, like getting a wheelchair for traversing long hospital corridors or asking for more covers to counteract the chilly combination of drafty rooms and skimpy johnny-gowns.

- If you are able to convey to healthcare workers that you are eager to help and collaborate with them as a partner in your loved one's care (and not just to criticize) then you will most often get a good reception. These days, most healthcare professionals are glad to deal with patients and caregivers who are active partners in their own care. The old days of the good patient being one who unquestioningly, blindly follows "doctor's orders" have been replaced by patients and caregivers who often show up armed with the products of their own extensive internet searches of remedies and resources. While these can be a burden and may contain errors, the basic idea that patients are taking responsibility for themselves makes the job of the professional easier. And you can be a part of this, advocating for your loved one, making sure that their priorities are being addressed.

Chapter 5: You Too Can Be a Website Manager

When David was diagnosed and began treatment, I anticipated the many, many calls I would need to answer from his many, many friends, and the prospect of having to repeat the same (painful) information over and over was daunting. Fortunately, I happened on an ad at the hospital for a free service for individuals to create their own interactive websites to communicate about a loved one's illness and treatment. I signed up right away and it quickly became an indispensable part of our action plan. Our website created a virtual community for us during a time of forced isolation; without it, life would have been not only super stressful, but also quite lonely. David summed up its importance in his entries on our website:

> *"... I hope you know that it is a great comfort to both of us that there are so many out there supporting, loving, praying. Cancer severely limits our time and energy for socializing – this is a virtual community, in the best sense. It is not as good as seeing people in person or speaking on the phone, but better than feeling isolated. Thanks." (August 2004).*

> *"Your messages mean a lot to us; our silence denotes only lack of energy and time, not lack of interest or lack of appreciation. Please know we are always not merely glad but thrilled to hear from you...We are very grateful for your continuing to communicate with us in spite of our silence. Your messages connect us with a world outside cancer, a world of healthfulness, business and optimism from which we sometimes feel removed." (March 2005).*

Our website served many very useful functions:

- It brought the world to us (virtually) so that well wishers could be present in our lives without interrupting us with visits or phone calls for which we might not have the energy.

124

- It was a vehicle for us to report on David's progress in as much detail as we wanted and to give clear explanations for the changes that we were observing.

- It displayed photos of us (on vacation, at family events, in the chemo suite at the hospital) to share our lives with others. I even made a graph of the changes in David's tumour marker and posted it on the site.

- It enabled us to solicit useful information, hints, and help from the many who logged on (as mentioned above, for example, when I was eager to make tuna tartare, which we believed might be good for David, I asked for and received recipes from several of our readers).

Since I was registered as the manager of our website, I was able to see the list of all the people who had logged on, even if they had chosen not to write a comment or message. And some days, when David felt particularly low, I would use this access to show him the list of all the friends and relatives who had logged on recently. He would be enormously encouraged to see concrete evidence of his virtual community, all the people who were thinking of him and wishing him well.

Some of our website entries were offbeat, almost whimsical, like this one from February 2005:

"a question about ear lobes.

Have any of you medical – or homeopathic or naturopathic or just plain curious – folks out there ever noticed sharp variations in ear lobe temperature (in yourself or a significant other)?

David and I are puzzled that at times when he is feeling particularly good his ear lobes are almost blazing hot; the converse is that when he is feeling low and lacking in energy, the lobes are very cool. I mean, I guess they are always 'cool', but you know what I mean ... We are eager to hear your thoughts on this."

Other entries were philosophical, spiritual, or even mundane (like my request for a recipe for tuna tartare). David found it very invigorating to compose messages for the website and to read replies; in November, 2003 he wrote:

"Writing to you my readers consumes me. I spend most of my time and energy thinking of what to say to you, rather than thinking of my nasty, volatile and aggressive mass. When we are communicating, I think, screw the cancer! So your reading this and getting back to me is no mere gesture; it underpins my resolve and resilience. Talking about your getting back to me, some of you have sent me humour emails surreptitiously to my private email address, but I do look forward to seeing your offerings on the website. ..Lisa and I plan for tomorrow as if I have no cancer, yet we fight the cancer every day in every way."

What You Can Do

- You can set up a website for free where you post messages and where friends and supporters invited by you can send you messages as well.

- On your website, you can send out bulletins about your loved one's condition/treatment, solicit help for you and for your loved one, post photos, etc.

- Your website can save you stress since it creates a virtual community of love and support without requiring you to undertake multiple interactions, phone calls, etc.: with one posted message you can communicate with many people at the same time, and you can offer them a chance to communicate with you in a way that they know won't inconvenience you or add stress to your already difficult days.

Why Is This Important?

- Being sick is a very lonely business; your website can restore a social life to both you and your loved one as you communicate with your virtual community.

- Wellwishers who are far away and in different time zones can read your postings and post their own messages of support at a time convenient for them, and you and your loved one can read them when it is convenient for you. A website also saves money since those who are far away can keep up to date on your loved one's condition and treatment without making long distance phone calls.

How to Do It

- If you have internet access (at home, at your public library, at a friend's) and if you can type with at least one finger, you can set up a website.

- You do not need to be a technical whiz to do this; there are a number of free websites available that will guide you through the process (The free service that I used to set up our website was Care Pages, http://www.carepages.com, which I found to be reliable and well designed).

- Your confidentiality is preserved since only those you invite to enter your website can read the messages posted there.

- You and your well-wishers can communicate in more than one language on your website if needed.

- There are many websites available. Some have extra bells and whistles, such as an interactive job and scheduling capacity for your volunteers to schedule their help (for related tips, see **6. Coordinator of Volunteers** below). See, for instance, www.caringbridge.org, www.thestatus.com, www.mylifeline.com, and www.tellthefamily.com. Many of these websites are affiliated with particular hospitals, but they are freestanding and independent. Hospitals affiliate with them both to benefit their patients and families and because it can add to the hospital's recognition (and perhaps to potential clients and/or donors). The websites differ from one another: shop around for the one whose features suit you best. There is even one for people seeking to build a community of people praying for a loved one (of any religion or creed): www.presspray.com.

- If you don't think you can manage a website, try to set up a "phone tree" among your well-wishers by providing information (or asking your question), which is then relayed to your supportive network by people calling one another.

Chapter 6: Coordinator of Volunteers

"Let me know if I can help," said our many relatives and lifelong friends; they said it frequently and they said it very sincerely. But each time, it felt like just one more burden: if they don't know what they can do to help, how can I organize them? I felt that many of our loving friends and family just didn't "get it." Here I was committing all my energies into fighting for David's survival every day, and their questions made me feel that I needed to help them. I knew in my head that they really wanted to help and just simply didn't know how, but for my part, I didn't have any extra mental energy left to help them help us.

And yet, wonderful things happened: Sidney, Stan, Bill, and Barry each drove David to and from treatment (a whole day commitment, during which they also engaged him in political debates, his favourite pastime). A huge pot of nourishing chicken soup arrived, as did many casseroles. Best of all, early on in David's illness, before the cancer had sadly wasted his face, Fred, an amateur photographer friend, took closeup photos of David beaming his famously big grin; he later delivered the enlarged, framed photos to my door, a wonderful gift I still treasure.

What You Can Do

- The people close to you, even though they may really want to help, may be unsure what to do or how to help you. And you may be too tired (or too distracted) to direct them. Instead of helping people help you, it may seem easier to just do it all yourself. But you want to save your energy for being with your loved one, a task where you are irreplaceable (See **Chapter 2: Being There**).

- There are those blessed people who just naturally seem to know what to do. They simply step right up to help and relieve you. But most of your friends and family probably feel awkward and scared (do people fear cancer could be contagious?), or they don't wish to impose. Many don't come forward because they feel it is respectful to wait to be asked. In these cases, you can help family and friends help you.

Why Is This Important?

- It really does take a village! As you have noticed by now, it is difficult being your loved one's caregiver all by yourself. If you have connections to others, now is the time you can really use their help. Don't be shy about calling in those I.O.U.s; if not now, when?

- Your friends do want to help you: make it easy for them! By telling your friends how to help you, you will actually be helping them as well. The giver usually gets more than he or she gives.

How to Do It

Below are some suggestions. You will want to add tasks that meet your particular needs.

- You may want to print your list and leave it for friends or email it to one friend who can then circulate it to others.

- Some technologically-inclined folks post such lists on a (password-protected) wiki-website so friends can sign up for jobs, trade visiting times, and so on.

Additional Considerations: Assigning and Coordinating Volunteers

- *Think of your own needs and how friends can spell you off.* Do you need time for yourself, a break from caregiving? Do you need to go out for a special meal or a concert so you can forget for a while your challenging caregiver job? Do you need someone to take over your usual daily/weekly tasks and commitments so that you can spend more time with your beloved patient?

- *Keep a list of everyone who offers to help you in any way.* Make sure you have their phone numbers and especially their e-mail (you can e-mail people at all sorts of hours, including when you can't sleep in the middle of the night). Coordinating volunteers is itself a very important volunteer job – and one that you should try to fill as quickly as possible.

Volunteer Coordinator Job Opportunities

Your volunteer coordinator can help with the following:

- Brainstorm about ways that people could help.

- Receive your list of help you need or jobs that you need done (organized according to a daily, weekly, or emergency basis). Your list can include any and all of your pre-caregiving tasks (for example, driving children to activities, picking up dry cleaning or groceries, cleaning, and so on) that could be done by a volunteer.

- Circulate updates and lists of jobs to concerned friends and relatives who will form your support network.

- Assign and coordinate volunteers to fill these jobs without duplicating and without adding to your burdens.

- Stay in email or phone contact with your network of concerned friends and relatives.

Volunteer Job Opportunities

- Driving your loved one to treatment, or being a back-up if the usual ride is unavailable.

- "Babysitting" your loved one, keeping them company so you can have some free time, get your hair done, go for a drink, or just meet a friend for coffee.

- Babysitting children, picking them up from school, driving them to activities, taking them out to a movie, to the park, etc.

- Shopping for groceries or other items, supervising service or trades people who come to do repairs at your home, etc.

- Phoning you and/or your loved one just to socialize and chat if and when that is appropriate. Socializing even by phone keeps you and your loved one connected to the outside world, giving you both respite from the illness. Our dearest friend Naomi would call on a regular basis and just leave a message, something like "you don't need to call me back; just want you to know I am thinking of you"; I loved receiving those messages, which made us feel less alone and didn't obligate us to even lift up a phone.

- Cooking (or buying) meals according to your list and taking into account any dietary restrictions.

- Lending or giving books, recorded music, humorous CDs, favourite DVDs.

132

- Using their particular skills, like hairstyling, manicure/pedicure, being a photographer of your journey, playing favourite tunes on guitar, carrying out household repairs, mending, sewing, gardening (this may include tending a flowering plant for the sick room), etc.

Chapter 7: Information Manager I: General Information ("Information is Power!")

His many years working in politics and in law had taught David the importance and power of information.

David was addicted to using three-ring binders (yes, those old-fashioned ones you may have used years ago to keep your high school notes in the pre-computer age); in these, he stored (literally!) a ton of information. The beauty of three-ring binders is that information can be easily added or removed, and it is all held securely; each binder covered one topic, with tabs for subtopics, making it easy to retrieve information as needed. The binders were arranged by topic, with a different coloured binder for each: white binders were for family history, blue for investments, yellow for travel ideas and plans, black for legal and tax information.

So we began a new series of binders for the cancer and coloured them red (for love? for war? for blood and guts? for urgency? Whatever the symbolism, it seemed right). We had a binder for "current newspaper articles and websites," for "treatment ideas," for prescriptions, lab tests and doctors' letters, and for "nutrition and cancer."

What You Can Do

- You can become "information central" for your loved one's disease and treatment. This can help you manage the journey and anticipate future developments.

- You need to actively pursue information; the newest research and information may not yet be common knowledge, even among healthcare professionals.

- Some important information may not yet have been published: information in medical textbooks tends to be about five years old, in journals about two years old, and presentations at meetings at least one year old. So it becomes extremely important for you to stay in close touch with people who specialize in the field to learn about the latest discoveries.

- Include fellow patients and their families: for David and me, some of the most useful information we were able to glean came from fellow patients and families.

- Another unexpectedly helpful source was daily newspapers, magazines, and online publications. These often had helpful nuggets of information in their health columns. Be aware, however, that such information must be checked against other, authorized sources for reliability and validity.

Why Is This Important?

- Information about your loved one's disease/condition will flow to you from TV and newspapers, from well meaning friends and relatives, and from the many caregivers you encounter.

- Make a note of all that you hear so that you can check one source of information against another.

- A piece of information may not be immediately useful, but you may need it at a later date; filing it away will make it available for you later.

- Once you have filed the information, you don't need to carry it around in your memory and you will be freer to take in new information.

- You may find that others approach you to ask for information; sharing what you know helps build a community of caregivers, a community that will benefit all involved.

How to Do It

- Get in the habit of scanning health columns in the media.

- Join associations devoted to your loved one's condition and attend their public events and support groups.

- Speak with fellow patients and caregivers as much as you are comfortable; there is a lot to be learned from others' experiences.

- Attend conferences, especially those relating to your loved one's condition and to caregiver issues.

- Store your information carefully: information is only useful to you if you can retrieve it when you need it.

- Note the date, source, and any contact details for each piece of information.

- Develop a filing system that works for you, so you can retrieve the information you have gathered. It can be anything from a series of electronic files on your computer, to the old-style paper file folders with scraps of information in them, to shoe boxes (with labels!) for different kinds and sources of information. The important thing is that you be able to retrieve and review the information when needed.

Chapter 8: Information Manager II: Information about Your Loved One's Condition and Treatment

One day, keeping David company in the chemotherapy suite, I sat near a woman writing furiously in a hardbound notebook as her loved one was being treated. Asked what she was writing, she said "I write everything down in this book; it's all here." I admired her determination and thoroughness, but while she may have experienced relief and a sense of control through her writing, she in fact had no way of retrieving any specific bit of information from her stream-of-consciousness record. As her notebook grew and grew, it became a cemetery for lost/dead information. How much better if she could have devised a way to access particular information when she needed it (what was last month's hemoglobin? what did the cardiologist recommend? what foods should we be avoiding?), and this information could have been extremely useful.

What You Can Do

- Many, many observations and bits of information from many sources are generated during a hospital patient's treatment, and that is why hospitals have developed the use of a chart for each patient stay. The physical chart has traditionally been kept in a three-ring notebook that is maintained in the hospital's Health Records department once you are discharged. Outside hospital, clinics and private offices are required to keep their own written records of your care. The information contained in all of these records (though not the actual paper it is written on) belongs to the patient; you are therefore entitled to request and receive copies of it. With these, you can create your own chart at home, as we will see below. Note: as I write this, computerization of hospital records here in Ontario is still uneven, and most health care facilities have some combination of paper and electronic records. All too often, you will still see nurses bent over pen and paper, recording observations at the end of their shift.

- It is important to remember that the law defines all the information related to your care as belonging to you. You can therefore request any of this information and your care provider must supply it. While it's amazing how many doctors are reluctant, say, to make a copy of blood or lab reports, patients are 100% entitled to these. You actually own this information; just ask for it. You may be charged a small fee, but the information is yours and you are entitled to it. And to repeat, information is power.

Why Is This Important?

The information you are compiling about your loved one's condition/treatment will have many uses, some of which follow:

- To recall the sequence of events and show you (and your healthcare professionals) the chronology of your loved one's illness/treatment.

- To fill in gaps for your healthcare professionals: all too often, information is not relayed from one professional to another in an accurate, timely way. Your documented information can be a great help to the treatment team.

- To facilitate your loved one's treatment in an emergency (when you are not likely to be in the facility where your records are kept).

- To enhance your credibility with healthcare professionals by showing up at medical appointments with your own chart.

- To help you understand what is going on and what you might expect in the future.

How to Do It

- Record one chronological log of events of your loved one's illness/treatment (on a calendar or in a notebook).

- In a separate place, record your questions (and answers received) and date them.

- These notes do not replace your journal of feelings; have your own private "Dear Diary" for these.

- List all contact people and their phone numbers, faxes, and e-mail addresses; list websites for resources such as Home Care.

- List all financial, insurance, legal, and tax information.

Most important of all, keep your own **chart** of your healthcare journey:

- Get in the habit of requesting reports of all your diagnostic tests, consultation notes, treatment summaries, etc. This information is legally yours and copies can be obtained from the Health Records department of the facility where you or your loved one were treated. Now what to do with all those papers? How to organize them? How to make sense of them? Sort your pile of documents out into categories, keeping a separate binder or section for each of the following:

Prescriptions

Keep a copy of each prescription, note who prescribed it and why, the date of prescription, and the drug's trade and generic names.

(NOTE: researchers generally refer to drugs by their generic names, and generic drugs cost less).

Results from laboratory tests

NOTE: whenever possible, try to go to the same lab so lab test results will be as comparable as possible, not contaminated by differences among laboratories.

Medical letters

Consultation reports, often written from a specialist doctor to your GP; these may be on file in the specialist's or GP's office.

Radiology and imaging reports

Many facilities will freely give you a CD of your radiology examination. You can also ask for and receive a copy of the crucially important report in which a radiologist describes and analyzes what was seen when you were X-rayed; you can get a copy of this radiologist note from your hospital chart.

Other healthcare professionals

Include information from social workers, physical therapists, nutritionists, and other allied health professionals.

Admission / discharge summaries

Prepared by the facility in which you or your loved one were treated, these give an overview of conditions, treatments, and results.

- Consider creating and laminating a one or two page summary of the key facts about your loved one's illness and care. (Since David's chemotherapy made his hemoglobin chronically quite low, the oncologist advised us to carry a letter from him explaining his condition, in case he ever had to be treated in the ER of a hospital that had no record of him. We printed this up, laminated it, and had it with us always in the trunk of the car.)

- A wallet-sized card listing all current medications can be very helpful as well.

NOTE: If keeping your own chart feels too onerous, try to have copies of all tests and diagnostic reports sent to your family doctor, who can coordinate the care your loved one receives from various caregivers.

Chapter 9: Going to the Beach
(Or, All Work and No Play Makes Jack a Dull Boy)

After being ill for a year and a half, with David well into his biweekly chemo treatments in New York, we both felt desperately in need of a holiday. The winter was grey, dark, and cold, and we started daydreaming about sunshine and beaches. How to escape? From dear friends Ted and Deanna, we heard of a beachfront condo available in Florida that we could book by the week. I booked us on direct flights, leaving after one chemo session and returning before the next, and daughter Naomi joined us there for a few days of sun and sand. We took all our medical equipment (for flushing his line, etc.) along with the usual holiday gear. David could not go swimming lest he infect his PICC line (the stump permanently inserted into his vein so that he could get I.V. treatments without having to have his veins punctured repeatedly). Some days, the Florida weather was cool, and some days, David spent a lot of time resting in bed, but still we felt we had been let out of jail. At the end of ten days, we returned refreshed for the next treatment. Photos show the joy we felt we captured.

What You Can Do

- You can be a combination personalized travel agent, trip planner and concierge, as well as being a loving caregiver.

- If travel by plane feels daunting, especially in these days of long airport waits and security checks, consider train travel, where you and your loved one can walk about during the journey.

- A day or a weekend at a friend's cottage can also be beneficial. "A change is as good as a rest," and it can do wonders for your spirits.

Why Is This Important?

- What you are going through is hard work, both physically and emotionally, and you (both) probably need a vacation.

- You will be part travel agent, part concierge, part go-fer, part loving caregiver.

- Does this seem like too much work? Feel it would be easier not to attempt it? Remember that you can task your volunteers with assembling your needed items and with making the necessary preparations for your holiday.

- And this may be your "new normal": cancer is fast emerging as a chronic illness and, as families dealing with chronic illness know, holidays and respite care are crucial to maintaining your strength and will to go on.

How to Do It

- Your travel itself needs to be preplanned: sacrifice spontaneity in order to best manage the needs of your loved one. Try to anticipate stresses and include backup measures. Below are some suggestions. Keep a list of what worked for you on your trip so that you can use the same strategies next time.

- Do request a wheelchair wherever and whenever possible! Among other advantages, it offers a way of transporting small luggage items and will get you priority in lineups.

- If you are planning a plane trip, try to anticipate how you will manage stressful delays; enlist the help of airline personnel. Do pack extra snacks and a water bottle (without water in it – you can fill the bottle after you have cleared the security at the gate). Give some thought too to managing the risk of infection (take face masks, sanitizers).

- If you are going by car, these are some things to take along (in addition to the usual tissues, bug spray, sunscreen, etc.):

  - A urinal or simple bottle for peeing if your loved one is male (David had an unforgettable episode caught in a highway traffic jam after hours of ingesting large volumes of fluid during chemotherapy),

  - Other toilet items, like Tucks or paper, hand disinfectant, and adult pads if using,

  - A hook for an I.V. to hang from the car's handrail (a coat hanger will work, in a pinch),

  - A blanket (if you don't already have one in the car),

  - Your usual safety material: flash lights, etc.,

  - A list of key phone numbers and email contact information,
  - Photocopies of prescriptions, phone numbers of pharmacies, etc.,

  - Nourishment: supplements like Ensure, soft drinks, juices, high protein snacks, favourite foods if eating is an issue,

- A (laminated) letter describing any special information for the ER in case you need to go there, including your MD's signature and contact information (see Chapter Eight),

- Distractions for you and for your loved one (magazines, books, DVDs, video games, favourite music CDs),

- Light reading material: a humour or thriller or something that grabs your (and your loved one's) attention

Chapter 10: Humour

As mentioned above, David and I were both very touched by the story of Norman Cousins who, gravely ill, had himself moved from the hospital to a hotel suite and, with the help of his Hollywood and television friends, spent all his days and evenings watching Marx Brothers and other movies, Candid Camera videos, and the like. He believes he laughed himself to wellness. And so David posted this RFP for Humour on our website:

"Governments and large companies initiate large projects by issuing Requests For Proposals. So, this is my Request For Humour. Many of you want to help and don't know how. Here is one tangible way. Say, once per week, send me the best joke you have heard that week. Please post it only to the website and not to my personal email, so that it will always be available to me, even months from now. A caution: quality is better than quantity, and brevity is good."

What You Can Do

- Not finding much to laugh about? At first glance, there may not seem to be a lot to giggle about in your situation, but look for the funny moments in this trying journey.

- Jokes in Cancerland? Yes, they really are there! Magnify them and share them with your loved one and with relatives and friends.

- Look for absurdity, perverseness, or irony in the healthcare system; if you look, you will find them all.

- In those moments where you feel you could either laugh or cry, try to laugh. It will do you both good.

Why Is This Important?

- Humour punctures dread, tension, and heavy moods. It is pretty hard to be sad or worried at the same time as you are cackling.

- Humour is life-giving; "laughter yoga" practitioners say it deepens breathing, enhances the body's own detoxification, fills the lungs with more oxygen, and expels more carbon dioxide.

- When sharing humour with your loved one, you will both experience a kind of togetherness that approaches your normal life.

How to Do It

- Be on the lookout for humour your loved one will appreciate.

- Use your website, listserve, or communication book to ask friends and family to supply humour.

- Since humour is very individual, tune in to what your loved one finds particularly funny and seek out videos, books, or audio tapes that will get a giggle.

- Try out a few different kinds of humour; don't be afraid to look silly.

- Keep refreshing your comic material.

Chapter 11: Making Meaning: Memories You Will Cherish

During our two and a half years in Cancerland battling David's cancer, there were many times when we manufactured occasions, like my 60th birthday when David and I took all of our family to a hotel for a wonderful weekend shared by those nearest and dearest to us. We had an agenda planned out in advance, with some activities and meals for the whole group, as well as some free time to pursue our individual interests. We took in the Ottawa Tulip Festival, had some delicious hotel and restaurant meals, and some of us even visited the nearby casino. The photos from that weekend show our warm relaxed moods as we sat in the sun or strolled near the tulips. And while I cannot forget that on our way home from Ottawa at the end of the weekend, David and I had to stop at every single highway rest stop to deal with his diarrhea, it is the memory of our whole family celebrating together that stays with me and warms me today.

What You Can Do

- Stop the rush of time by planning and implementing events, however small, that will be meaningful to you and your loved one.

- Creating and capturing your own meaningful moments will give you and your loved one a chance to triumph over the illness.

Why Is This Important

- The mundane, day-to-day drudgery of illness and caregiving can swallow up your days (and nights) and leave little energy for special occasions. However, if you can muster the energy to plan and execute special occasions (or ask some of your volunteer helpers to do so), then you will be extremely glad later: those are the memories that will stay with you and sustain you.

- You will not remember each time your loved one was too exhausted to do anything but sit around or lie down, nor will you recall each drive to the hospital or clinic, each sponge bath, or each injection, but you will remember the joy of celebrating together with those closest to you in the middle of your "war." Whatever the outcome, these memories will warm you.

- Focusing on a pleasurable event interrupts the train of morbid thoughts that can take over your mind and home if you haven't something better to put in its place.

How to Do It

- You can plan occasions that will have particular meaning for you and your loved one: surprise visits, sporting events, social gatherings, special meals, all within the constraints of your loved one's illness and the limited energy you each have.

- Start small: a pleasant, meaningful half-hour enjoyed by your loved one with friends or family can be enormously helpful in changing their mood and yours.

- Ask your volunteers to plan and facilitate arrangements for these occasions (planning, driving, inviting, and so on). If your volunteers are not available for such tasks, consider hiring professional helpers to make such events happen.

- Photograph and record these occasions so you can relive them together later. Consider posting your photos on your website (see **Chapter 5: You Too Can Be a Website Manager** above).

The best recourse against illness is living well. You and your loved one will benefit greatly when you take control of your lives even under the shadow of illness.